Praise for *Raising Awe-Seekers*

"Deborah Farmer Kris's urgently needed book, *Raising Awe-Seekers,* offers an inspiring roadmap for bringing more awe into your children's lives and for finding more awe as the caregiver that you are. In this age of anxiety, there is nothing more important for caregivers to do, and no better path than reading this book."

— **Dacher Keltner,** professor of psychology at UC Berkeley, author of *Awe: The Science of Everyday Wonder and How It Can Transform Your Life*

"In *Raising Awe-Seekers,* Deborah Farmer Kris reminds us that childhood and parenting aren't just about the daily routines, extracurriculars, sporting events, and appointments that take up so much time and mental energy. She shows us how one of the most enjoyable parts of life is awe and explains many simple ways to spark awe for ourselves and our children. This book is a masterpiece in showing parents how to set an example for their children that awe is a necessary part of living a life filled with joy, curiosity, and wonder."

— **Afsaneh Moradian,** author of the Jamie Is Jamie picture book series

"Deborah Farmer Kris's first parenting book couldn't come at a better moment. At a time when life feels overwhelming and the future seems more uncertain than ever, *Raising Awe-Seekers* is the perfect antidote to the confusion, anxiety, and stress we're all facing. The perspective and practice of wonder is overlooked and underappreciated, and yet it is precisely what every single one of us needs in order to remain hopeful, engaged, compassionate, and resilient. This book is a fantastic read, and the suggested practices are reasonable, doable, and—best of all—fun! I cannot recommend this book highly enough for every parent human out there."

— **Carla Naumburg, Ph.D., LICSW,** author of *How to Stop Losing Your Sh*t with Your Kids*

"*Raising Awe-Seekers* is a transformative guide that reminds us of the profound role awe and wonder play in nurturing resilience and connection in our children. Deborah Farmer Kris masterfully weaves personal stories and research to show how fostering a sense of belonging, kindness, and curiosity can strengthen the bond between parents and children. This book beautifully captures the essence of intentional parenting, inspiring us to slow down, embrace the little wonders, and cultivate a joyful family culture. It's a must-read for anyone looking to deepen their relationship with their child while helping them thrive in an ever-complex world."

— **Bryana Kappadakunnel,** author of *Parent Yourself First*

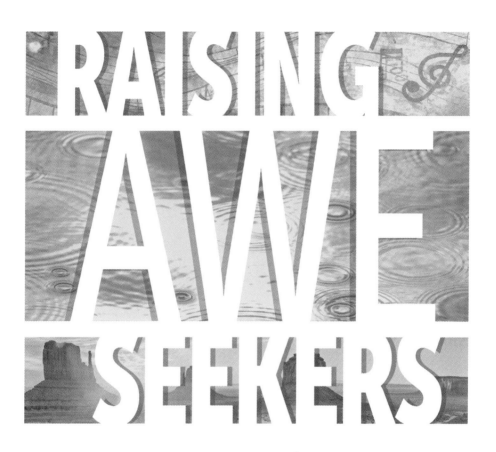

RAISING AWE SEEKERS

How the Science of Wonder Helps Our Kids Thrive

Deborah Farmer Kris

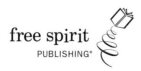

free spirit
PUBLISHING®

Library of Congress Cataloging-in-Publication Data
This book has been filed with the Library of Congress.
LCCN: 2024049996

Free Spirit Publishing does not have control over or assume responsibility for author or third-party websites and their content. At the time of this book's publication, all facts and figures cited within are the most current available. All telephone numbers, addresses, and website URLs are accurate and active; all publications, organizations, websites, and other resources exist as described in this book; and all have been verified as of November 2024. If you find an error or believe that a resource listed here is not as described, please contact Free Spirit Publishing.

"Sometimes" by Mary Oliver (p. vi) is reprinted by the permission of The Charlotte Sheedy Literary Agency as agent for the author. Copyright © 2008, 2017 by Mary Oliver with permission of Bill Reichblum. | Portions of "Nature and Attention" (page 29) were adapted from "Age of Distraction" by Deborah Farmer Kris published in *Deseret Magazine* and are used with permission. | The author's interview with Susan Cain (page 158) and portions of "Needing to Be Needed" (page 119), "How Parents Can Confront the Crisis of Kindness" (page 182), and "Finding the Helpers" (page 173) were previously published as "How to Help Kids and Teens Process Bittersweet Feelings," "Why Kindness and Emotional Literacy Matter in Raising Kids," and "The Benefits of Raising Hopeful Kids in Cynical Times," respectively, by Deborah Farmer Kris on *MindShift*/KQED and are used with permission. | Portions of "Belonging Looks Different for Tweens and Teens" (page 121), "The Difference Between Noise and Sound (and Why It Matters)" (page 45), "Making Room for Hobbies" (page 105), "Coaching Tweens Through the Interference" (page 185), and "Better Thinking Through Nature" (page 52) are adapted from articles by the author previously published on *MindShift*/KQED and are used with permission. | Portions of "Becoming the Helpers" (page 180), "Helping Kids Navigate Loss" (page 152), "Post-Traumatic Growth" (page 156), and "Needing to Be Needed" (page 119) are adapted from articles by the author originally published on PBS KIDS for Parents and are used with permission.

Edited by Cassie Labriola-Sitzman
Cover and interior design by Courtenay Fletcher

Printed by: 68348
Printed in: USA
PO#: 15631

Free Spirit Publishing
An imprint of Teacher Created Materials
9850 51st Avenue North, Suite 100
Minneapolis, MN 55442
(612) 338-2068
help4kids@freespirit.com
freespirit.com

FSC
www.fsc.org
MIX
Paper | Supporting
responsible forestry
FSC® C005010

To MK, AK, JK & CK—
you are the wonders of my world.

Instructions for living a life:
Pay attention.
Be astonished.
Tell about it.
—Mary Oliver

CONTENTS

Introduction 1

1. The Wonder of Nature 17

2. The Wonder of Music 43

3. The Wonder of Art 65

4. The Wonder of Big Questions 87

5. The Wonder of Belonging 115

6. The Wonder of the Circle of Life 141

7. The Wonder of Human Kindness 167

Afterword 195

Acknowledgments 198
Notes 200
Index 216
Reading Guide 227
About the Author 231

INTRODUCTION

Childhoods rich with awe are good for the child.
—*Dacher Keltner*

On an August night, my dad shook me awake at 2 a.m. I stumbled out of bed and into the backyard. Dad—a taciturn geneticist who felt more at home in a lab than at a party—had already spread out a large quilt for me and my four older siblings. A couple of the kids had not responded favorably to the wake-up call and were still in bed. Those of us who had lay there in grumpy silence.

But then, a streak of light sliced through the sky. And another.

"Woah!"

"Over there!"

"Look at that one!"

For hours, until pink light washed away the stars, my siblings and I lay on our backs, mesmerized by the cosmic dance of the Perseids. My nine-year-old self would have described the night as *awesome*—an apt choice, since within the word is its emotional correlate: awe.

Rediscovering Awe

Nothing fascinates me more than child development—how kids learn, develop social and emotional skills, and form habits that will help them thrive. This passion has sustained me through two decades as a K–12 teacher and administrator, parent educator, child development

1

specialist, and education journalist. And I have two amazing kids who, of course, test every theory I've ever had about child development.

And *yet*, for all my training and practical experience, I'd overlooked a key concept—one that boosts children's mental and emotional well-being, strengthens their social ties, and supports their curiosity and internal motivation. I was missing the thing that had infused my own childhood with meaning and joy. I was missing *awe*. Or rather, I was feeling it without naming it and yearning for more without knowing why. And I had no notion of the compelling body of research that underpins this three-letter word.

That changed in September 2021.

A school had reached out, asking for a parent presentation on "resilience and stress management." Resilience is crucial to psychological strength, and it's a topic I normally enjoy presenting on for parents, but I just couldn't muster my usual excitement. For a year and a half, since the start of a global pandemic, it seemed like all my articles and workshops had been focused on how to help kids and adults "navigate these unprecedented times." I knew my parent readers and workshop attendees were looking for this advice—I was too. As parents, we'd shouldered our own anxiety while helping our kids work through a massive upheaval, including the loss of routines, anticipated milestones, and the security of normalcy. We'd risen to the task again and again and again. That's what parents do, after all. But I was tired, and the other parents I knew were tired too.

Staring at this school's email invitation, I froze up. *I don't want to talk about stress and resilience again*, I thought. *I want to talk about . . . hope.* But what would that look like?

That same week, I was finishing edits on my picture book *You Wonder All the Time*, which celebrates young children's innate curiosity. Somehow, I stumbled upon a forty-five-page white paper called "The Science of Awe" from the Greater Good Science Center at the University of California, Berkeley. The paper summarized fifteen years of research, much of it research from the Center's founding director, Dacher Keltner.

Sitting at my computer, reading the research on awe for the first time, I got goosebumps. I remember how the light filtered in through the office window as I read. My brain whirred, connecting these findings with decades of child development research. I laughed, scribbled notes, and texted the paper to a dozen friends and colleagues. I was awestruck.

Over the next several weeks, I devoured every article and academic paper I could find on the benefits of awe and wonder. And then I called Keltner to interview him for a *Washington Post* article about how parents can help their kids experience these emotions. In the days that followed the article's publication, I watched the response from readers. Scores of parents, educators, and faith leaders shared the piece. It made the rounds in online groups. Awe seemed to be resonating with everyone.

Researching awe has changed my life. It has affected how I take my daily walks, what I listen to in the car, and how I think about my daily schedule. When the dog wakes me up at 4:30 a.m. to go out, I am less inclined to grumble and more likely to look up at the stars. Becoming an awe-seeker is even (slowly) improving my attitude toward New England winters. Most importantly, awe has influenced my parenting in profound and concrete ways. And I believe that understanding this emotion can change your life and your parenting too.

Raising kids has never been an easy job. In addition to tending to their basic needs, as parents we must contend with the many challenges facing our children and teens: intense pressure to achieve, the hazards of social media and the online world, struggles with focus and motivation, spiking rates of anxiety and disordered eating, and worries about climate change, political strife, global crises, and local injustices, to name just a few. There are wonderful parenting books out there that give pinpointed insights and advice on each of these topics. This book offers something a little different. It aims to reorient you and your parenting toward something fundamentally human: the capacity to wonder.

This book is about raising awe-seekers and becoming one yourself.

What Is Awe, Exactly?

Before we continue, take a minute or so and make a list of all the human emotions you can think of. When I ask parents and kids to do this exercise, they usually respond with variants of four basic emotions: happy, sad, mad, and scared. Our brains also go quickly to excitement, frustration, fear, anger, joy, and worry. But in all my years of giving workshops on children's emotional development, I have yet to have a participant write *awe* on their list.

So, what is awe?

Awe is perhaps our most overlooked and undervalued emotion. It is what we feel when we encounter something vast, wondrous, or beyond our ordinary frame of reference. It evokes a sense of mystery, reverence, or wonder. It is the feeling that washes over us when we hear a beautiful song, watch a flock of geese fly south, or see images from the new NASA telescope.[1]

Keltner, who has spent two decades studying this emotion, describes three ways you might know you are experiencing awe: tears, chills, and "whoa."[2] For example:

  | Think of a moment when you watched your child do something beautiful, and your eyes got misty (tears).

  | Think of a time you heard a song or a story on the radio, or read a passage of text, that gave you goosebumps (chills).

  | Think of a time when you saw a stunning sunset or vista that prompted you to utter, "Wow!" (whoa).

For kids especially, I would add this: wide eyes. I love seeing a young child's eyes pop with amazement when they encounter something brand new—like a chicken hatching out of an egg, an ocean wave, a parade, a street performer, or a baking-soda-and-vinegar volcano. As Keltner writes, we can all find "the extraordinary in the ordinary . . . the wonders of life are so often nearby."[3]

Why Does Awe Matter?

If you take an evolutionary view of human development, emotions serve distinct purposes. Fear keeps us alert for dangers and prepares us to deal with them. Prolonged stress isn't healthy, but short-term stress can be our friend: It gets us ready to act, it reminds us of what is important to us and worth protecting, and it can heighten our senses and provide us with crucial information we can use to keep ourselves and others safe. I remember the first time my son saw the ocean at age two and strode right in. Luckily, my stress was operating at proportional levels to his nonchalance, and I used that burst of adrenaline to race in to get him.

Likewise, anger, with reason and limits, can prompt us to protect others and to confront injustice. Loneliness reminds us that we all crave companionship. Disgust keeps us from eating the chicken in the fridge that doesn't smell right. Contentment and joy send us powerful signals about what replenishes our bodies and spirits and helps us find equilibrium.

So what's the purpose of awe? Why do we get goosebumps when we watch Simone Biles vault herself into the air or catch our breath when we see a rainbow after a storm? How does this emotion help the human species survive and thrive?

For such an overlooked emotion, awe packs a punch. According to the research I outline in this book, awe supports our physical, mental, and emotional well-being. It strengthens curiosity and humility and enhances our connection to other humans. Several studies you'll read about describe how experiencing awe can make us kinder and more generous—prompting people to work cooperatively, share resources, and sacrifice for the common good. These types of behaviors and dispositions strengthen family and community life today and likely helped our early ancestors survive.[4] In addition, awe has been linked to improved mental well-being, including a decrease in PTSD symptoms and a reduction in biomarkers of inflammation.[5] As a bonus, feeling awe also supports academic engagement, because this feeling spurs curiosity about the world, strengthening internal motivation.[6]

Put simply, awe supports just about every outcome that we want for our kids, our families, and ourselves:

- Do we want our kids to be compassionate and civic-minded?

- Do we want to form healthy and meaningful relationships?

- Do we want our kids to retain their innate curiosity as they grow and strengthen their motivation to learn?

- Do we want everyone in the family to develop perspective, resilience, and the capacity to find wonder in everyday life?

Awe supports all these aims. And yet it's an emotion that, generally speaking, we and our children do not experience enough.

In Keltner's *Awe: The New Science of Everyday Wonder and How It Can Transform Your Life*, there is one paragraph that I highlighted, underlined, and starred (my annotating trifecta):[7]

One of the most alarming trends in the lives of children today is the disappearance of awe. We are not giving them enough opportunities to experience and discover the wonders of life. Art and music classes do not make the school budget. The free-form play of recess and lunchtime is being replaced with drills to boost scores on tests that have only a modest relation to how well kids do in school. Teachers must teach to those tests rather than engage students in open-ended questioning and discovery, where the unknown is the centerpiece of the lesson. Every minute is scheduled. And the natural world children are experiencing is undergoing mass extinctions. It's no wonder that stress, anxiety, depression, shame, eating disorders, and self-harm are on the rise for young people. They are awe-deprived.

With pediatric health experts raising the alarm about the mental health of children and teens, helping our kids experience a little more awe could become part of our collective response. As Keltner puts it, "One simple prescription can have transformative effects: Look for more daily experiences of awe. . . . Their benefits are profound."[8]

How Do Kids Understand Awe?

But do kids really feel—and understand the feeling of—awe? And how early in life can they recognize it? It's not one of the core four emotions (happy, sad, mad, scared) that we usually talk about with young children. In 2023, researchers at the University of Chicago conducted a study with children ages four to nine. They found that children can discern awe-inspiring experiences from other kinds of experiences. Researchers wrote: "[Children] perceive diverse positive effects of awe-inspiring experiences—in terms of their motivation to explore, awareness of things to understand, and multiple aspects of their sense of self. . . . Our work provides evidence that awe-inspiring experiences, such as seeing nature's beauties and power, are readily appreciated even from an early age."[9]

Fan Yang was the lead researcher on this project. She is the director of the Human Nature and Potentials Lab at the University of Chicago, which researches human happiness, meaning, and awe. She told me that she hopes her research will help parents see that "children are capable of experiencing much more and appreciating the world in deeper ways."

I can confirm just how accurate Yang's reflections are. Recently, I visited a school to read my picture book *You Have Feelings All the Time* to a large group of kindergartners. Before opening the book, we generated a list of emotions they already knew. The children quickly moved beyond happy, sad, mad, and scared—calling out feelings such as grateful, frustrated, surprised, exhausted, worried, and hopeful. How did they develop this sophisticated emotional vocabulary? They had to first experience these emotions themselves, and then they needed guidance in finding a name for what they were feeling. Identifying feelings gives children a mental framework for their emotional world— and it helps them identify emotions that they *want* to experience. When we seek out awe with our children, and give them a name for the feeling, we help bend their worlds toward wonder. They can choose to become awe-seekers, with us and on their own.

While writing this book, I spoke to hundreds of kids and teens about awe and wonder, through classroom visits, school assemblies, workshops, and personal conversations. While *awe* was largely a new word for these audiences, I found that kids—even preschoolers—could grasp its meaning. Kindergartners loved to tell me their favorite "wow facts." When I asked a group of nine- to twelve-year-olds, "What do you think *awe* means?" hands shot up. A fourth grader said, "It's like when you really look up to someone—you are in awe of them." A classmate added, "It's when you want to say, *Wow! That's so cool!*" Fifth and sixth graders offered these synonyms: *flabbergasted, amazed, dumbstruck, surprised*, and (my personal favorite) *transfixed*. After a visit to a high school in Massachusetts, the newly elected student government chose "Awe" as the theme for the upcoming school year. I have had teenagers reach out to me weeks after a presentation to ask me the name of the song I played or the painting I showed. Kids and teens have also eagerly shared their own stories about what it felt like to dance in *The Nutcracker*, learn about the Franklin Expedition, meet a red-tailed hawk, create art, sing with friends, lead a drum circle, hold a new baby, or experience a parent's supportive love. And, with their permission, I've included many of these stories in the pages that follow.

Where Do We Find Awe?

The best part about awe is how accessible it is. How *ordinary*. We don't have to take our kids to the Grand Canyon to experience it. Awe is an everyday emotion, something we can feel during a morning walk, a puppy playdate, a bedtime story, or a soccer game.

How do we know this? Researchers Yang Bai, Maria Monroy, and Dacher Keltner collected awe stories from adults living in twenty-six countries. They drew from a diverse pool: members of all major religions, people living in democratic and authoritarian countries, and people with widely varying educational, socioeconomic, and cultural backgrounds.

Participants were given a definition of awe and then asked to share a time when they felt this emotion. Researchers then coded the 2,600 responses, looking for patterns in people's awe-inspiring experiences. They identified several sources of awe. This book is structured around seven of the main sources,[10] with an eye toward how each relates to parenting and child development.

1. **Nature:** From sunsets to ocean waves to the first spring flower, nature is a universally accessible source of awe. And, as I discuss in chapter 1, there are tangible benefits to getting our families outside and in touch with the natural world.

2. **Music:** For humans, song is our first language. We react to our babies' coos and cries; they respond to our lullabies and sing-song voices. For teens and adults, a meaningful piece of music can elicit intense emotion, and a song from childhood can transport us back in time. Auditory wonders, and how we can use them to support kids' development, are covered in chapter 2.

3. **Art:** This broad category includes making art, seeing art, and experiencing the wonders of design—such as looking up at a

skyscraper or walking into an artfully designed courtyard. Chapter 3 dives into the visual world, sharing ways parents and kids can experience art together.

4. **Big Questions:** Think of the last time you read a book, listened to a podcast, or learned something new that made you sit up and say, "Wow." Chapter 4 explores how packed childhood is with this source of awe as kids seek answers to compelling questions—and how we can join them.

5. **Collective Effervescence:** This is the energy that comes from being part of a group that is working toward a common purpose. Most kids crave this source of awe—it's why they join sports teams, drama troupes, and D&D clubs. Chapter 5 is about belonging and how we can support our kids' desire to be part of a larger whole.

6. **The Circle of Life:** Think about how you responded to your child when they were a baby. Did your face brighten as you tried to make them smile or marveled at their tiny toes? Think, too, of the reverence and mystery that can surround a loss. Chapter 6 explores how awe can help us reframe how we talk to kids about life and death.

7. **Human Kindness:** The most common source of awe is witnessing other people's goodness. Moral virtue is inspiring. "It's kindness and courage," Keltner told me. "We really have this capacity to be moved by other people." That's the topic for chapter 7.

This is not a prescriptive parenting book. Rather, in these pages, you'll encounter research and hear from experts in various fields about how their work relates to parenting and wonder. You'll learn about the benefits of awe and ways to make awe-seeking intentional. I share stories from parents and kids, as well as my own stories (with my children's permission) about living and parenting as an awe-seeker, in hopes of inspiring you to invite more of this emotion into your and your children's lives. Finally, each chapter offers concrete ideas and resources—from activities to book lists—to help you fill your kids' worlds with wonder.

Parenting Anchors

Before we dive into the heart of this book, I want to share four broad concepts that anchor my approach to parenting and that you'll find infused throughout these pages. I have been writing about these ideas for years. But when I began to study awe, I quickly realized that these concepts also support awe-seeking. So as you read the research and encounter new ideas in this book, think back to these anchors and how you might infuse them into your parenting.

1. Slow Down Childhood

Today's highly structured, competition-oriented child-rearing culture largely ignores or even stifles awe. Waking hours are often filled with adult-directed activities, pressures, or obligations. That leaves kids less time to wonder, wander, or tune in to their emotions and surroundings. As Keltner told me, awe requires unstructured time: "How do you find awe? You slow things down."

I've worked with fourth graders who were so programmed with after-school classes and weekend activities that they rarely had time to play. I've spoken with eighth graders who told me they "don't have time" for hobbies and activities that bring them joy. I've worked with stressed-out, sleep-deprived high school juniors and seniors for whom activities were—first and foremost—résumé builders for college admissions. Awe requires being present in the moment, and that's not easy in a future-oriented, go-go-go culture.

Pressing the pause button to make more room for awe will likely take some adjustment. I think about all the times I've barked at my kids to hustle while they were, say, crouched on the sidewalk, staring at a dandelion growing through a crack. But when I think about my favorite parenting moments, and hear from other parents about theirs, they are often centered around simple moments of awe: wandering through the park with my kids, watching fireworks on a hill, or snuggling together during a thunderstorm. It's the joy that comes from seeing your child's eyes grow wide with understanding, watching your kid who struggles with nerves perform confidently on stage, or noticing siblings be good to one another.

2. Embrace PDF

As a mental model, I love the acronym PDF, developed by Stanford University's Challenge Success, an organization focused on "strategies that improve well-being, engagement, and belonging for all K–12 students." PDF stands for:[11]

Playtime
Downtime
Family time

Challenge Success founder Denise Pope says the research is clear: "Every kid needs PDF every day."[12] Awe fits beautifully into this paradigm. Wonder is often playful. Wonder requires downtime. And wonder can strengthen family relationships as you get curious *together*.

Of the three, adults and kids struggle most with downtime. When we don't have an activity, agenda, or digital distraction, sometimes we don't know what to do with ourselves. That's why I'm a big believer in the generative power of boredom. Within seconds of finishing screen time, my son invariably says, "What can I do, Mom? I'm bored." Sometimes I give him options, but he usually swats them down reflexively. Other times I respond: "Brilliance is born of boredom."

I'm not saying my son *likes* that response, which is one that both my kids have heard countless times, but it's a gentle tease with a deeper meaning. As kids wrestle through the uncomfortable feelings of not knowing what to do in the moment, they (usually) find their way. They become curious and creative out of necessity, pulling out a craft or making up a game, picking up a sketchpad or concocting some "potion" from jars in the spice cabinet. Questions lead to more questions. Wonder begets wonder.

3. Practice Radical Curiosity

As a parent educator, I sometimes field the question *So, what's your best advice?* It's an unanswerable query because there is no single checklist for raising kids. But parents can never go wrong with this: curiosity. Get curious about who your kid is. Get curious about what motivates them and confuses them. Get curious about why your teen is acting the way they are. Get curious about what your kids are curious about.

Robert Waldinger has made it his life's work to study what it means to live a "good life." He directs the Harvard Study of Adult Development, which, for more than eighty years, has followed the lives of 724 participants and more than 1,300 of their descendants. He detailed the results in his book with Marc Schulz, *The Good Life: Lessons from the World's Longest Scientific Study of Happiness*. I had a chance to talk to Waldinger, and when I asked him what wisdom his research held for parents, he offered up the concept of "radical curiosity." He defined this as a "real, deep curiosity about what others are experiencing."

To practice radical curiosity, Waldinger says, look at one person in your life and ask: *What's here about this person that I haven't noticed before?* Your answer could "be anything," he said, "even the way sweat forms on your partner's forehead." Radical curiosity can transform family relationships because "we get lulled into the assumption [that] *Oh, I know this person. I know how they're going to react.*" Curiosity allows a relationship to grow as the people within it grow and change.[13]

Take our kids. When they are newborns, we are hyperaware of every sigh, smile, and cry. When they are toddlers, we note each milestone.

Years later, do we respond to our eight-year-olds' meltdowns with the same curiosity? The middle school brain develops more rapidly than at any age except birth to age three: Are we awestruck by our eleven-year-olds' cognitive leaps? Are we curious about what makes our eleventh graders giggle like five-year-olds? As I hope you'll see time and again as you make your way through this book, one of the most readily available sources of wonder for parents is the child right in front of us.

4. Become an Awe-Seeker Yourself

I can't begin this book without stating an obvious truth, and it's one I need to tell myself repeatedly: Our kids take their cues from us. They are astute anthropologists of human behavior and tend to imitate what they see. So if we want them to feel more awe, we must become awe-seekers first. If we want them to experience wonder, we must open ourselves to it too.

The phrase *be a lifelong learner* is so overused it's almost meaningless. So let's reframe it: What if we paid more attention to what piques our curiosity? What if we tuned in to our tears, chills, and whoas? And then, what if we named those things out loud to our kids? When we get excited about a new skill we're learning, pause to savor a favorite song, experiment with a new recipe, marvel at a sunset, or investigate a nest in a tree, we remind the kids watching us that wonder is a lifelong pursuit.

One of the best ways to feel collective family awe is this: Listen to kids' questions and notice what brings them wonder. When we notice what makes our kids say *wow*—what gives them goosebumps or expands their minds in beautiful ways—we learn more about who they are right now and who they might become. When we pay attention to our kids' sources of awe, we validate their experiences and invite them to keep exploring.

Parenting is always a push-pull. We push kids to develop healthy habits and skills, to try new things, and to discover their interests. They push back, pulling us in unexpected directions on their path of self-discovery. Together, we grow. It's messy, *wonder*-ful, and *awe*-some work.

I remember dragging my kids on an autumn hike, perhaps trying to channel my nature-loving dad. Like I did at their age, they grumbled a bit. But after an hour of scrambling over rocks, kicking leaves, and watching herons stalk prey, one of them turned to me and said, "Next time I don't want to come, please remind me of this feeling."

I can, because that feeling has a name. And this book is all about it.

CHAPTER ONE

THE WONDER OF NATURE

A child's world is fresh and new and beautiful, full of wonder and excitement. . . . If I had influence with the good fairy . . . I should ask that her gift to each child in the world be a sense of wonder so indestructible that it would last throughout life."
—Rachel Carson

Awe doesn't often make the headlines. But on April 9, 2024, the front page of *The New York Times* read, "A Divided America Agrees on One Thing: The Eclipse Was Awesome."

Though our town was about three hours south of the path of totality for that solar eclipse, a celebratory atmosphere permeated the community. The day before the eclipse, local online groups were overrun with residents hunting for eclipse glasses and others offering up their extras for free. One of my kids spent the afternoon constructing a moveable 3D eclipse model while the other built a pinhole camera. Many schools let out early. Libraries and community groups hosted watch parties.

My family kept it simple and put out lawn chairs and blankets in the front yard. Neighbors wandered over to join us, and a gaggle of kids climbed our Japanese maple tree to get closer to the sun. The birds went silent as we craned our necks toward the sky. As *The New York Times* reported, "For this moment, a wide swath of this country did the same thing, together, happily and in wonder. Our world of divisions and distractions—of TikTok and politics and disasters—fell away, leaving us quiet with our breath held in awe."[1]

Back in 2017, as the United States was getting ready for another solar eclipse, I had the chance to interview NASA scientist Amy Mainzer for PBS KIDS. (Your kids might know her as Astronomer Amy from the show *Ready Jet Go!*) I thought of her words as I watched the moon swallow up the sun. "Eclipses offer us a powerful reminder of our place in the cosmos as we go about our daily lives," she told me. "We sit on a small planet speeding around a gigantic sun, whirling through the galaxy."[2] That's what awe does: It reorients our perspective, reminding us of how small we are in the scheme of things. And despite our culture's emphasis on celebrity and status, a healthy sense of "smallness" can be just what our kids need.

A Few Things We Know About Nature, Kids, and Awe

Not surprisingly, people name nature as a key source of awe. Since awe involves encountering something vast, then oceans, sunsets, thunderstorms, stretches of desert, and fields of flowers are awe-inspiring by definition.

But our kids don't need awesome vistas to find wonder in the natural world. And kids often do more to pull their parents toward nature than the other way around. When my kids were four and seven, I wrote this about their relationship with the outdoors:

> As the spring days grow longer, my kids resist going to bed. Who can blame them? Bugs and birds are far more appealing than bath and bedtime. Everything they see sparks their wonder: ants swarming a dead beetle, bees drinking from flowers, plants pushing up through sidewalk cracks, peeper frogs croaking, dragonflies perching, and wild turkeys strutting down the street.

They want to dig in the dirt, climb trees, blow on dandelions, and hunt for four-leaf clovers.

As parents, our challenge is less about getting our kids to enjoy nature, and more about how to slow down and make time to experience the natural world together—and how to help our kids keep that connection as they grow into adolescence and beyond.

The documented benefits of getting outside for kids of all ages are legion. Time in nature supports cognitive development, stress reduction, creativity, focus, mental and physical health, social skills, gross motor skills, and environmental awareness.[3] Simply put, time outside makes kids healthier and happier in a host of ways.

Here's a fun fact: Did you know that the presence of greenery *outside* a school building may support the academic performance of students learning *inside* it? A study of Massachusetts elementary schools showed a relationship between the "greenness" of a school's environs and schoolwide academic performance. How did researchers measure this? Every spring in Massachusetts, students take the MCAS, a series of standardized tests. Using satellite images, researchers measured the vegetation levels around each school during testing season. They also adjusted the testing data to control for other demographics—things like family income level, student/teacher ratio, and attendance rates. In the end, they found that "results showed a consistently positive significant association between the greenness of the school in the Spring . . . and schoolwide performance on both English and Math tests, *even after adjustment for socioeconomic factors and urban residency*"[4] (emphasis added).

Here's a less-fun fact: Today's kids spend more time inside than any previous generation did. That's largely related to technology. According to a 2021 report from Common Sense Media, American tweens (eight- to twelve-year-olds) spend an average of five-and-a-half hours each day on screens, and teens are on screens for an average of eight-and-a-half hours daily.[5] In one study, 65 percent of US American parents surveyed reported playing outside every day during their childhood—but only 30 percent of their children do the same today.[6]

Nature is a readily available, yet underutilized, source of awe for our kids. As awe researcher Dacher Keltner writes, "It is hard to imagine a single thing you can do that is better for your body and mind than finding awe outdoors."[7]

Nature, Awe, and Mental Health

Psychologist Craig Anderson has spent years exploring the connection between awe and mental health.[8] His studies don't just take place in a lab. As part of his research at the University of California, Berkeley, Anderson embarked on over a dozen white water rafting trips. And he took two types of study participants with him. The first group included young adult veterans who had experienced combat missions. The second group included teens from underserved communities who had been exposed to community violence. These teens "reported higher levels of [PTSD] symptoms than our veterans did," Anderson told me.

Anderson's team found that experiencing awe in nature predicted improved well-being in both groups. A week after the rafting trips, participants self-reported a 30 percent decrease in their PTSD symptoms. They also felt less stress and got along better with friends and family. Lab tests corroborated these perceptions. In comparing before-and-after saliva samples, researchers found that this intensive, nature-based experience reduced participants' stress hormones and inflammatory markers.[9]

One of the rafting participants was a college-age combat veteran. In a video about his experience on the trip, this young man noted that when he gets together with other veterans at a bar or social gathering, they usually ended up reminiscing about their time in the military, "almost like we're stuck in it." But when he went rafting with other young veterans, they were so absorbed in the sights, sounds, and emotions of the moment that "we ended up never talking about combat—I felt like we were all really living in the moment."[10]

When I talked to Anderson about those rafting trips, his enthusiasm for the potential of this research was palpable. He often paused while speaking, as if in recalling these moments in nature, he was reexperiencing the accompanying awe. But it would be "a shame if the only way we could get those benefits was by going white water rafting," he said. So, in a second study, Anderson's team asked college students to record positive experiences they had during their normal lives over a two-week period.[11] His team then went back and coded which positive experiences included being in nature, "things like, *oh, I took a few minutes to relax on the quad* or *I noticed that the flowers in North Berkeley were particularly gorgeous that day*." Here's what they found: Students who "spent time in nature on a given day felt more satisfied with life that evening than those who didn't" and, building on this pattern, "students who spent more days in nature over the two weeks saw greater improvements in well-being during that time."[12] Anderson summarized it this way for me: The more that students "had these everyday experiences of nature, the more awe they felt and the better well-being they showed at the end of that two-week period." Anderson said that he envisions a day when doctors prescribe time outdoors as a concurrent, complementary mental health treatment: "The awe that we feel in the outdoors could be a useful part of our health care system."

What's the application for parenting? Anderson's research leads me to this question: If time in nature can measurably improve the mental health of young people, and especially those who have experienced combat and community violence, could regularly taking our kids outside serve as a protective measure? Could time in nature strengthen our kids' abilities to withstand life's stressors?

Plenty of researchers have established a relationship between nature and mental health. A study from the Medical College of Wisconsin found that "higher levels of neighborhood green space were associated with significantly lower levels of symptomology for depression, anxiety, and stress," after controlling for a wide range of factors.[13] The researchers concluded that "greening up" our neighborhoods could be a relatively low-cost, high-result "mental health improvement." And this isn't just true for urban areas. Scientists at Cornell University looked at how access to nature influenced the mental health of children living in rural areas. They found that nature acts as a buffer: "Specifically, the impact of life stress was lower among children with high levels of nearby nature than among those with little nearby nature."[14] And a 2024 NIH study found that young children (ages two to five) who lived near dense green spaces, such as parks or forests, had fewer symptoms of anxiety and depression.[15] According to the lead scientist, "Our research supports existing evidence that being in nature is good for kids. It also suggests that the early childhood years are a crucial time for exposure to green spaces."[16]

I love the concept of nature as a "buffer." Nature might not protect our kids from challenges, but perhaps the awe they experience in it can build a protective barrier, improving their mental health and allowing them to navigate life just a bit more easily.

Hattie's Story

Hattie Ransom is a wildlife biology major at the University of Montana and a self-proclaimed "bird nerd." She shares how nature helped her navigate adolescence.

I'm grateful that my parents encouraged me from a young age to get outside and create a relationship with nature, including my love for birds. Looking back, I can see that my bird journey truly provided me a safe space and a creative outlet growing up.

The first time I remember really noticing a bird and wanting to know more was when I was ten. There is a creek by my childhood home, and I would play there all the time. I remember setting up a camp chair and pulling out an old pair of binoculars I had found in the closet. I saw these birds that were just so beautiful. My mom got me a little bird book, so I flipped through it and found what I was seeing: a flock of cedar waxwings. That's when I remember my love of birds starting.

When I was twelve, I met a woman at my aunt's wedding who happened to be a bird "bander" at the University of Utah. She let me come to their banding station. There wasn't much I could do, but I got to hang around, be the "bird bag girl," and observe the whole process. I loved it, even when I had to get up at 4 a.m. on a summer morning.

In high school, I struggled a lot with mental health, and sometimes I had a hard time feeling connected with my peers because of it. I often felt lonely. One day, I was walking on a trail near my house and found a red-tailed hawk's nest. After that, when I was in a negative head space, I would take a spotting scope and go watch the hawks. I loved watching the hawk parents as they took care of their kids. Nature is very grounding for me.

One thing I love about birding is that you can do it anywhere. There's not a lot of gear you need—just a pair of binoculars and maybe a guidebook. There are birds anywhere you go, even in big cities. It can be like a treasure hunt! Once you see a bird and try to ID it, you suddenly realize how many birds are out there! The diversity is incredible.

Nature and Generosity

The more I talk to other parents, the more I believe that all parents' hopes for our kids are quite similar and surprisingly simple. We want to raise kids who are kind and brave—young people who can form meaningful relationships and who are attuned to the greater good.

In chapter 7, we will look at the wonder that comes from witnessing human kindness. But first, here's a preview, via the flip side of that: Feeling awe can prompt us to be kinder. Awe orients us toward others because it reduces our focus on the self.

Paul Piff is currently a psychology professor at the University of California, Irvine, but he did his graduate research out of the University of California, Berkeley. While there, Piff and his colleagues at Berkeley devised two studies to investigate whether nature can increase prosocial—or helpful—behavior. In the first, one group of participants watched video footage of magnified water droplets moving in slow motion. A second group watched a less inspiring video. Both groups were then tasked with dividing up resources to share with others. The water-droplet group showed more fairness in this task than their counterparts did.[17]

As Piff shared in an article for *Greater Good Magazine*, "Even these minute droplets remind you of the intricacy and complexity of the natural world, and in so doing bring about feelings of awe and the small self. And that is one of the remarkable qualities of awe. You don't have to climb a huge mountain and take in a grand view to feel it."[18]

In another study, Piff's team took the participants outside the lab.[19] The Berkeley campus boasts a towering grove of eucalyptus trees. Researchers asked one set of participants to stand and gaze at the soaring trees. The other participants stood in the same spot but were told to direct their gaze at the back of the campus science building—a nondescript brick structure.

After a participant had spent some time staring at one view or the other, a stranger walked by, stumbling and dropping their pens to the ground. This stranger was part of the research team, but the participants did not know this. You can probably guess the result: The tree-gazing participants picked up more pens than their building-gazing counterparts. They noticed. They helped. Instead of focusing inward, they reached outward.

More than any other study, this tree-gazing experiment fascinates people when I give presentations about awe. I wonder if it's partly because of the implicit metaphor within: Two people—standing in the *exact* same place—can feel uninspired or awestruck depending on where they direct their gaze.

We can't always choose the spot we stand in—literally or metaphorically. One of the most painful truths of parenting is just how much is out of our control. We worry when our kids worry. We hurt when they hurt. And while we can't (and shouldn't) fix every woe, we can choose where we "direct our gaze" and how we help our kids view the situations they find themselves in. Are we focused on the brick wall, or can we expand our view to see the trees that surround us? Time in nature can help reframe our perceptions, renew our resilience, and reach out to others with kindness and generosity.

Nature and Mental Chatter

One aspect of wellness kids *and* adults wrestle with is something called *mental chatter*. Chatter is the voice in your head that runs through your fears, worries, and to-dos. It is the racing thoughts that wake you up at 4 a.m. and remind you of the thoughtless remark you made last week or the words you and your tween exchanged in anger. It's the judgmental voice that compares your parenting to sparkling Instagram Superparents. It is the looping images of monsters under the bed that keep your four-year-old from falling asleep or the worries that keep your teen's brain spinning late into the night. We all experience mental chatter, and it can be overwhelming.[20]

Adolescents are wired for inward focus and social comparison, so their inner voices can be particularly loud. That's why, when I read *Chatter: The Voice in Our Head, Why It Matters, and How to Harness It* by Ethan Kross, my first thought was, *How do we get this information to tweens and teens?* Kross is a psychologist and neuroscientist, and he has spent years studying this inner voice. When I spoke with Kross, he expressed the same desire to get this info into young people's hands. In fact, he told me that at the end of a college seminar on this topic, one of his students raised her hand and asked, "Why didn't I learn about this earlier? This would have been really useful when I was in high school."

"When chatter consumes our attention, it leaves little left over to do other things, including managing our feelings," Kross told me. "Chatter zooms us in on the problem. We engage in a tunnel-vision way of thinking." I'm sure you can think of a time when you were so worried about a situation at work or upset about a conflict with a friend, parent, or partner that you had a hard time focusing on anything else. For kids and parents who are troubled by their inner voices, Kross wants them to know that's "totally normal" and that "there are tools you can use to manage how you engage with that voice." According to Kross's research, any strategy that allows a person to zoom out can help quiet the mental noise. Going outside is one of those strategies.

Time in nature is a powerful tool to zoom out because the awe we find there helps us broaden our perspective, Kross told me. "You feel smaller when you're contemplating something vast and indescribable—and when you feel smaller, so does your chatter." He points to the pictures NASA has released from the James Webb Space Telescope. "Every dot is a galaxy. It's mind-blowing. In comparison, how consequential is the chatter I experienced earlier today because my daughter and I got into a little argument about cleaning up the house? Multiple galaxies or the condition of the living room?" Nature-based awe offers us the gift of perspective and humility. There's nothing like the night sky to remind you that you are a minuscule part of an expansive universe. That humility can be liberating.

Here's a trick I learned from my teaching days. If I had a student or advisee who felt stuck in their concerns about schoolwork or social life, I would often take our conversation outside—to a picnic table on campus grounds or on a walk around the perimeter of the building. Just moving from inside to outside seemed to help stressed-out kids relax, breathe easier, and get more creative in their problem-solving.

That insight has helped me with my own kids as well. I will often pull them outside to walk the dog with me when I notice their mood spiraling. Is it easy to get them outside when they are upset? Not always. But it is one of the best tools for emotional regulation I've found. In fact, walking outside has been my favorite form of self-care since I was a teenager. When I was a young mom, these walks involved pushing two kids in a stroller. Now they usually include my dog—but they *also* include more watching and listening than ever before because I've learned how to take "awe walks."

Awe Walks and Forest Bathing

The great naturalist Rachel Carson encourages us to approach nature with the wonder of toddlers and the wisdom of elders: "One way to open your eyes to unnoticed beauty is to ask yourself, 'What if I had never seen this before? What if I knew I would never see it again?'"[21] What if I had never seen a red-tailed hawk before—how would that feel? What if I knew that I would never see a daffodil again?

Though she wasn't writing about awe walks specifically, Carson's advice can be a guide. An awe walk involves purposefully turning your attention outward, looking and listening for things that inspire awe—like a towering cloud formation or the sound of crunching leaves. According to a 2020 study, older adults who took weekly fifteen-minute awe walks for eight weeks reported increased positive emotions and less distress in their daily lives.[22] I have taken an awe walk nearly every day since reading this study. My phone stays in my pocket and my headphones out of my ears so that I can, as Carson advises, deliberately look and listen for beauty.

Aran Levasseur, a high school teacher at San Domenico School in California, was inspired by the research around awe walks and wanted to bring it to his students. Would his current tenth graders—tech-savvy digital natives—discover the same sense of wonder that elders had on these walks? Over the course of the year, the students took walks and created "Almanacs of Awe." As Levasseur wrote in an article for *Greater Good Magazine*:[23]

> For some students, it was the beauty of nature that captured their attention. A "butterfly's many subtle colors were revealed the more I observed it," wrote one student. "The stillness of the butterfly made me feel at peace." For another, "seeing the way the water trickled and the way the light fractured and rippled on the rocks underneath amazed me. It felt like looking at art." A humble pumpkin was a source of awe for a different student: "This pumpkin gave me awe because it is crazy to me how something so complex can be grown with just a seed, water, and sun."

I loved this reflection from one of the teens, which captures the healthy humility that comes from spending time in nature: "I felt awe when I went under this redwood tree and looked up at its branches. In the moment I looked up at the tree, it seemed never-ending. I think the tree had me in awe because it was so much larger than myself and gave me a sense of perspective."

While the term *awe walk* may be new to you, perhaps you've heard of *forest bathing*—or *shinrin-yoku* in Japanese. The term was coined by Qing Li, a professor at Nippon Medical School in Tokyo and president of the Japanese Society of Forest Medicine. In his 2018 book, *Forest Bathing: How Trees Can Help You Find Health and Happiness*, Li describes how spending time in nature can lower blood pressure, boost immune systems, and reduce stress hormone levels in the body. And in an article published in *Environmental Health and Preventative Medicine*, Li writes that forest bathing is "not exercise, or hiking, or jogging." Instead, he says, "It is simply being in nature, connecting with it through our sense of sight, hearing, taste, smell, and touch."[24]

Writing about forest bathing reminds me of one of the most gifted educators I have met. Molly James is a kindergarten teacher in New Jersey. Last summer, she watched a short video about the artist Vicki Thomas called "Fascinated by Nature." In the video, Thomas says, "If I had a tombstone, it would have on it, *Vicki, who always said, 'Oh, look!'* because that's what I'm always doing."[25]

James laughed in recognition. "Oh, look!" is also her go-to phrase when she hikes. That got her thinking about the five- and six-year-olds in her care. What if they started taking "Oh, Look!" walks around campus? "Oh, look" is such a simple, accessible phrase, and one young kids already use: "Oh, look, Mom—a centipede!" "Look! There's an airplane in the sky!" "Look, Dad, a puddle! Can I jump in it?" (My kids often remind me to "look up" when my face is turned down, staring at my phone.) James said that when she takes "Oh, Look!" walks with her class, "We first look for big things, and then little things. We come to notice the small wonders and the value of taking a second look." These second looks help us realize that, as Thomas says, "If you look at a plant, you're not just looking at a plant, you're looking at life."[26]

> "I had never really paid much attention to sunsets. But one night as I sat on a beach watching the sun set, something changed. I thought, *Wow, this is really nice, being here on the beach watching the sun melt into a million different shades of pink and orange, while hearing the waves crash on the surface.*"
> —Kate, high schooler

Nature and Attention

In my twenty-five years working in the child development realm, I have never heard so much dismay about the inability to focus as I have in the last four years. Mostly from parents. Talking about themselves.

Has it ever been so hard for kids, teens, and adults to pay attention? And how can we help our kids learn to focus when we struggle to do so ourselves?

Attention is the ability to direct our limited mental resources when and where we need them. The key word here is *limited*. Attention is a finite cognitive resource. It can help to think of it like a battery that is drained by overstimulation, multitasking, worry, internal chatter, distraction, pings, and dings.

Sometimes, I can barely write a paragraph without becoming distracted by a police siren, a push notification, or a text from my spouse. I'll suddenly remember that my son didn't put on sunscreen before camp or that I need to pick up milk for tomorrow's breakfast. Ugh, I have to pay the electricity bill and schedule dental check-ups for the kids. Did I ever Venmo the room parent for the teacher gift? Remember to text Grandma to see how the appointment went? Why, why, why do we have to sign up for summer camps in November?! When was the last time the dog was groomed? How do I have sixty-seven unread emails? What was I writing about again?

When my brain is distracted, bird listening is one of my favorite tools. Not birdwatching, bird *listening*. My kids and I stumbled upon this strategy by accident.

In mid-March 2020, the ambient noise of planes, cars, and trucks disappeared in an instant. At the time, I was teaching high school, my husband was a middle school administrator, and my kids were both in elementary school. Our house was filled with sounds from four different online schools, and the inside of my head was exploding with anxiety.

But the neighborhood was erupting with birdsong.

My son's online kindergarten experience was not going well. His teacher was amazing, but five-year-olds just aren't built for Zoom. One day, he crawled under his blankets and flat-out refused to log on. He needed a break, but I needed him occupied during my classes. So I downloaded an app called Merlin from the Cornell Lab of Ornithology. This free app "listens" to birds and identifies them for you.

The app appealed to my kid's insatiable interest in animal facts. That morning, and many subsequent ones, he took a tablet into the backyard, pressed a button, and walked around listening to birds. He watched in delight as the screen filled with the names and images of the birds who (like him) got up with the sun. He hunted in the branches for the bird that matched the call. When he returned indoors, I noticed he could focus better on his morning lessons.

His wonder got me hooked too. I began to notice patterns: the birds who stay all year, those who return in the summer, and those travelers who pass through on their migration routes. For most of my life, birdsong was nothing more than white noise. In listening with awe, however, I've found myself brought to tears by the call of a song sparrow or a lark. When my brain gets noisy and distracted, tuning into the sounds of nature calms it down faster than meditation.

Ethan Kross helped me understand why an activity such as bird listening is so helpful—especially when we are feeling overwhelmed and distracted. Specifically, he introduced me to the term *attention restoration theory (ART)*. ART suggests that the sights and sounds of nature are not just enjoyable, they can also charge our attention battery.[27] Studies show that kids and adults can focus more effectively after spending time outside. Nature is a cognitive tool "hidden in plain sight," Kross told me, because "nature restores attention."

So how does it work? "When you go for a walk in a green space, you are surrounded by stimulating sights like trees and bushes and flowers. They capture your attention, but they do so in a very soft and gentle way," said Kross. This is sometimes called "effortless attention" or "soft fascination." Nature stimulates the brain without taxing it, restoring our capacity to focus. "When you leave the walk," he said, "those attentional resources are more refreshed for thinking carefully about the problem that you're grappling with."

Kross told me that even looking at pictures of nature scenes can be restorative: "I have changed the way that I walk to work, and I've changed the way I decorated my office based on this work."

We all know what it's like to feel attentionally tapped-out, distracted by headlines, deadlines, overflowing inboxes, and the endless practical minutiae that comes with raising kids. We also know that if our kids need *one* thing from us, it's our attention—not constant hovering, but at least a few minutes a day of undistracted, positive attention. No multitasking. Phone down. Doing something that fills them up without interjecting: *So what's your homework tonight? Did you put your clothes away? Don't forget to . . .*

This might look like picking dandelions with a toddler or playing a round of catch with your kid in the backyard. Last night for me, this looked like a short evening walk with my middle school daughter. Suddenly, our dog found a frog in the yard, and we just stood there, laughing and enjoying the frog's hops and our pup's playful pounces under the stars.

Better Thinking Through Nature

"Daydreaming is good for you," I told a group of eighth graders. They looked at me skeptically. Isn't that what they are told *not* to do by parents and teachers? You know, "Quit daydreaming and focus."

"If you want to be creative, you have to let your mind wander sometimes," I continued. "Have you ever had an awesome insight or new idea while you were taking a shower, staring out a window, or lying on the grass? These 'aha' moments don't always happen while you are focusing. When I have writer's block, I know it's time to take a walk."

According to Annie Murphy Paul, author of *The Extended Mind: The Power of Thinking Outside the Brain*, humans did not evolve to do their best work while sitting down inside. In Paul's research, she met a common theme in the writings of many influential scholars: They did their best thinking while walking outdoors. The philosopher Henry David Thoreau wrote, "The moment my legs begin to move, my thoughts begin to flow." Novelist Virginia Woolf penned an essay about how her imagination came alive while walking the winter streets of London. Poet William Wordsworth would carry a pencil and journal with him and walk for hours in the countryside, sometimes purposefully getting lost.[28] I can imagine the awe he felt, stumbling upon unexpected beauty, as he records in the poem "I Wandered Lonely as a Cloud":

> I wandered as lonely as a cloud
> That floats on high o'er vales and hills,
> When all at once I saw a crowd,
> A host, of golden daffodils;
> Beside the lake, beneath the trees,
> Fluttering and dancing in the breeze.

Our everyday language reflects this instinctive understanding about creativity. Paul told me, "We say we are 'stuck' or 'in a rut' because we have this idea that stasis and nonmovement do not promote creativity. And then when we are thinking creatively, we say we are 'on a roll' or our thoughts are 'flowing.'"

For a more modern context than Wordsworth, look at this study: Stanford students were told to complete creative tasks—such as coming up with unexpected uses for a paper clip. Creative output increased by an average of 60 percent when walking instead of sitting down.[29] And yet how many of our kids and teens think that in order to be productive they must sit at a desk and muscle through? What if we recognized a walk outside or time on a swing as a way to rejuvenate the brain and inspire creative thinking?

Wendy Suzuki, a neuroscientist who studies the effects of exercise on the brain, says that outdoor playtime has cascading benefits for children. She told me, "It really has to do with what we know about how the brain works and how we can rejuvenate brain activity—particularly focus, attention, and mood. When you cut down [outdoor play], you are removing time that kids can run around. And when they run around, their brains are getting a bubble bath of good neurochemicals, neurotransmitters, and endorphins. These help memory and mood. A simple burst of exercise helps students focus better."[30]

Outside time can also help our kids when they are struggling with how to solve a problem. Michael Roberto is a professor of management at Bryant University and author of the book *Unlocking Creativity*. If we want to be more creative, he said, "sometimes we need some distance from the problem we are trying to solve." Roberto told me that he is a proponent of "wandering outside." When we wander, we are doing something outside of our routine. Our children's days are often incredibly routine—from the morning routine, to the daily school schedule, to the predictable evening activities, to the bedtime routine. Obviously, routines are important, but when we do something spontaneous—like exploring a new park or a new neighborhood in the city—Roberto says we are more likely to "spot something novel, and novelty spurs the brain; seeing incredible creations sparks our own minds to develop original ideas."

Roberto even recommended not overprogramming family trips, leaving downtime in order to make room for novelty. He was speaking right to me. I am a planner. Recently, we traveled to California for the first time as a family. In the days leading up to the trip, I had carefully scripted the week's itinerary, and that itinerary took us to an aquarium at 1 p.m. on a Monday afternoon.

When we arrived, right on schedule, the place was teeming with school groups. You had to walk sideways just to make it through the lobby. One of my kids doesn't love big crowds, and we all realized quickly that it was time to go. However, that left a big hole in the schedule before dinner. We decided to go explore a nearby beach trail. We didn't know what to expect, so when we stumbled upon slumbering sea lions and a cliffside of cormorants, we gaped in astonishment. Soon my kids were exploring tide pools and naming the sea lions and making up silly stories about them. It was one of the best types of creativity: creating memories.

Nature Onscreen

As I combed through the studies about awe and nature, something struck me: Not many of the studies actually took participants outside. Most involved showing the experimental group awe-provoking videos and images of nature, such as clips from the BBC's *Planet Earth* series.

This led me to wonder: *Can screens replace nature?* If you made it through this chapter, I think you know that screens won't ever *supplant* the awe we feel in nature. But accessing nature through screens can be a *supplemental* source of wonder.

Because of this, I now project a beautiful landscape on the screen as people walk into my classes or workshops. I follow nature photographers and Earth artists on Instagram. And I've found that the more I choose to follow these types of accounts, the more the app's algorithm works in my favor, changing the tenor of my feed—the make-up tips and celebrity gossip replaced by images of sand art, cherry blossoms, and ridiculously beautiful birds.

Inspired by these photos, I started a practice I call "something beautiful every day." This is usually a photograph I take on one of my walks, but sometimes it's a song or a story or a poem. About the same time I started this practice, a friend's child was diagnosed with cancer. Susanna was *that friend* when I was in high school. When I felt like I was split into pieces—morphing into whoever I thought a teacher, parent, coach, or peer wanted me to be—Susanna seemed to see it all and love all of me. But now we live a thousand miles apart, and I couldn't even bring over dinner to ease her family's burden. So I decided to text her my "something beautiful" moment a few times a week. No need to respond, just a regular tether to an old friendship during a painful and overwhelming time.

Sometimes I text my daughter the same photos, songs, or goosebump-and-wow-inducing reel. And guess what? My kid will send me back art, photos, and adorable reels of ducks and possums. I underestimated how valuable this medium of communication would be for our parent-child relationship—these daily windows into what we each find wonderful.

All that said, the question of screens and awe is complicated. Keltner told me that screens usually serve as a "gateway to awe rather than a direct experience of it." They can help us find artists, musicians, and places we might not otherwise discover. Films such as Louie Schwartzberg's *Fantastic Fungi* allow viewers to see the natural world in a way that wouldn't be possible without technology. That's a helpful way to think about tech like the bird listening app: It's a tool that augmented my son's fascination with birds.

But we also need to remember that most of the apps we use are not designed to make us feel awe, Craig Anderson told me. Nor do they prioritize our well-being. Instead, "they're designed to keep us in front of the app." In addition, the social-evaluative nature of social media can be at cross-purposes with the healthy "smallness" that comes with awe. If you want to feel the benefits of "noticing things like the flowers blooming or the light filtering through the leaves on the trees," Anderson says, "your attention can't be wrapped up in a phone."

Where do I land? I believe educator Maria Montessori said it best when she wrote, "There is no description, no image in any book that is capable of replacing the sight of real trees, and all the life to be found around them, in a real forest. Something emanates from those trees which speaks to the soul, something no book, no museum is capable of giving."[31]

A Final Thought

In 2011, I gave birth to my first child and planted my first garden. At the time, we were living in North Texas—a place with two short growing seasons interrupted by a stretch of summer heat where only peppers and cucumbers seemed to flourish. I really didn't know what I was doing when I planted in July. Mothering and gardening—I struggled to figure out both that first year. As I wrote in an essay in July 2012, somehow that garden ended up nurturing both me and my daughter:

> Tomorrow is her first birthday, and she hasn't gotten a fire ant bite yet. That's something of a miracle, given the menacing mounds that keep popping up in our backyard.
>
> We just got back from a trip to see family, and though the neighbor boy did a great job watering, I have skeletal sunflowers to hack down, tomatoes to trim back, weeds to pull, oversized cucumbers to pick, and fire ants to kill. And mosquitos. One of our flower boxes didn't drain properly, leaving a breeding pool for the blood-suckers. The baby (almost toddler) is dotted with red bumps.
>
> It's 7 a.m., and we have already been to the park and back, pushing out the door before sunrise to enjoy a couple hours of fresh air before the heat puts us in house arrest. I'm stuffing dead leaves into the composter, and she's crawling off her blanket toward the flower bed. She won't touch a cucumber, but she'll devour handfuls of dirt and munch on clovers.
>
> I started the herb and flower garden the month before this child was born, digging out a rocky bed (and keeping that detail away from my doctor). The first vegetables went in the raised planters when she was one month old. It was late August, and for the first time since age four, I was not starting school. That's seventeen years as a student and thirteen years as a teacher. I wanted this child, but it was painful to let go of the structure of my entire

conscious life. She kicked in her bouncy seat while I planted lavender beneath the pear tree and thinned the irises. She watched as we took out two diseased peach trees and replaced them with roses. She teethed on fresh carrots and chard.

When the first frost hit, she watched me from her blanket bundle as I draped the tomatoes in flannel sheets, desperate to save hundreds of green fruits that had felt my postpartum nurturing. I may have cried when some did not survive the night.

We started seedlings together inside in January: spring peas, spinach, radishes, dill. By the time we placed them in the earth in early March, she was crawling and smearing her face with soil. At the garden store, I would show her two flowers and let her point. She favors purples and yellows, just like her mama.

I like to think I've tamed this yard, but every time I plant something new, I add to its wildness. The squash becomes a home for potato bugs. The tomatoes attract masses of birds that stalk me as I lay foil and drape netting. The composter draws flies. And now the mosquitos and fire ants, which come out to play in the hours when it is finally cool enough to sit outside.

I like that my daughter has spent her first year this way. I like that we both have constant dirt beneath our nails. I don't garden out of any sense of "should." There are enough *shoulds* that haunt me as a parent. This was an invitation. Something in this little plot of earth asked me if it could be a part of our family and invited me to be a part of hers. Sometimes I think Mother Earth was looking out for this new mom, inviting me to learn something about how things grow.

5 Wonderful Ways
to Get into Nature with Kids

1. The Story of a Tree. Choose a tree to investigate up close. What kind of tree is it? What shape are its leaves? Where are the tree's seeds: in a pod, pinecone, nut, or fruit? Look for evidence of other living things using the tree for their home, such as a nibbled leaf, nests, or holes that might double as a creature's home. Visit the same tree several times over a year and make note of the changes it goes through. What does it look like in each season? What differences does your child notice? Take or draw pictures to document the changes.

2. Nature Journaling. Blank notebooks invite wonder. Kids of any age may enjoy keeping a nature journal. Independently or with your help, they could record their questions, jot down observations, and sketch things they see outside.

3. Moon Watching. In the evening or early morning, go outside with your child and find the moon in the sky. Introduce simple moon vocabulary: Is it a new moon? A crescent moon? A quarter moon? A full moon? For a full cycle, take a trip outside each night to see how the moon is changing. Bonus: Take a picture of the moon each day and compile the pictures into an art project or slideshow.

4. Nature in Your Community. You don't need a special trip to the mountains or beach to help your kids experience the wonders of nature. Go on a family walk and follow your kids' pace as they stop to dig in the dirt, jump in leaves, or hunt for treasures. Explore a local farm, city park, or Audubon center. Go to an open field to observe the night sky. Turn over stones to see what creatures live beneath. Find the animals and trees that live in your neighborhood. Notice the changing light and shadows. Plant something—anything—and watch it grow.

5. Five Senses. When you are outside with children, play the five senses game. Ask:

- What do you see?
- What do you hear?
- What do you smell?
- What could you taste?
- What textures can you feel?

10 Awe-Inspiring Picture Books About Nature

In the Small, Small Pond **by Denise Fleming.** This book is a great introduction to pond life for preschoolers and toddlers. Vibrant, magnified pictures of insects and animals are paired with peppy verbs such as *wiggle, jiggle, waddle, wade, swoop,* and *swirl.*

Tree: A Peek-Through Picture Book **by Britta Teckentrup.** Studying a tree is a great way to investigate seasons and animal habitats. As you turn each page, the scene changes slightly. My kids love pointing out which animals have appeared or disappeared and how the branches, buds, and leaves are shifting.

How to Bird **by Rasha Hamid.** Birding is a wonder-filled activity that anyone can do. Featuring the skyline and natural spaces of New York City, this book invites children to explore birdwatching, with each page featuring a new birding strategy.

Because of an Acorn **by Lola M. Schaefer, Adam Schaefer, and Frann Preston-Gannon.** This beautiful book, with its simple text, is a great introduction to our ecosystem and the circle of life. Because of an acorn, a tree grows; because of a tree, a bird has a place to build a nest, and so on. The next time your child finds an acorn outside, they will have a whole new appreciation for it.

Redwoods **by Jason Chin.** A young boy on the subway finds a book about redwood trees—and finds himself magically transported to a California forest. You get to peak over his shoulder and read his book along with him, learning from text and pictures about these natural wonders. It might inspire you to ask questions about trees in your corner of the world. What are their names? How old are they?

The Street Beneath My Feet **by Charlotte Guillain and Yuval Zommer.** What nature can you find on a city street? This fold-out book takes you down, down, down below the sidewalk—from pipes to animal burrows to rock layers to Earth's core. This is the kind of book that you lay out on the floor and explore over and over again.

Up in the Garden and Down in the Dirt and *Over and Under the Pond* **by Kate Messner and Christopher Silas Neal.** These two books pair exquisite illustrations with informative text—introducing kids to pond and garden ecosystems. What's happening above ground and above the water? And what is happening underground and under the surface?

Jayden's Impossible Garden **by Mélina Mangal and Ken Daley.** Jayden sees nature everywhere in his neighborhood: in the acorns and rocks, the birds and squirrels, the sun and snow. When his mom tells him, "There's no nature in the middle of the city," he takes it as a challenge. With the help of an elder in his building, Jayden creates a community garden to show off all the things that can live and grow in the city.

Look and Be Grateful **by Tomie dePaola.** Rather than listing reasons to be grateful, this simple book by the legendary Tomie dePaola reminds the reader to pay attention: to look, listen, and notice the beauty in the world around them. The beautiful illustrations include a boy studying a ladybug and sharing fruit with his sister. As the text reminds us, "Today is today, and it is a gift."

Maps **by Aleksandra Mizielińska and Daniel Mizieliński.** It's a short name for a big book. This oversized illustrated guide to every continent has provided my son with hours (and hours) of fascination. He got it as a present when he was three. Five years later, it is still a favorite—an endless scavenger hunt for cities, rivers, mountains, animals, plants, and cultural tidbits. Never underestimate the power of a map to inspire wonder!

CHAPTER TWO

THE WONDER OF MUSIC

*Music makes us want to live. You don't know how many times
people have told me that they'd been down . . . But then a special
song caught their ear and that helped give them renewed strength.
That's the power music has.*

—Mary J. Blige

A few years ago, we adopted a puppy—Cupid—an adorable fluffball
who was (and is) a bit anxious. On one of his first car rides, Cupid
began to tremble and whimper. One of my kids, distressed at our pup's
distress, had this idea: "Try singing to him, Mom."

I began to hum "Baby Mine," the lullaby I sang to my children
every night for years. It's what I sang when they woke up to thunder
at 3 a.m. It's what I sang when they were sick and needed soothing.
Sometimes, I hum it to myself as a calming strategy. As I sang in the
car, Cupid began to settle down in the same way I'd seen my kids settle
into sleep.

"Song is our very first language," music educator Anita Collins told
me. "It is an incredible mechanism to connect with babies and other
human beings." And the occasional puppy, it seems. Collins, author of
*The Music Advantage: How Music Helps Your Child Develop, Learn, and
Thrive*, said that when you sing to babies and young children, "they
are picking up that you are a safe person, that you are a person they
are connected to." Don't worry about the quality of your voice, she said.
"Your baby doesn't care. You are your baby's favorite rock star." When

my kids were four and six, I asked them, "I wonder when you will stop wanting lullabies every night." The six-year-old responded, "You can stop three days before my eighteenth birthday. I'll need a few days to get used to it before I head to college, but it'll be hard." The four-year-old said simply, "When I'm forty."

A study on awe and children found that engaging with music and art has "powerful effects" on children's emotions: "Infants as young as five months are more likely to smile and rhythmically move their body parts in response to music by Mozart than to baby talk, and six-month-old infants are transfixed more by their mother's singing than by her speaking."[1]

It's not surprising, then, that people around the world identify music as one of their top sources of awe. After stumbling upon a song posted by cellist Yo-Yo Ma on social media, my friend Tracy wrote, "Serious question: What is it about music? What happens in our bodies when we listen to a cello (or any music) [that] will make us stop like a deer in a glen—and why am I weeping at 6 a.m. in my kitchen?"[2]

Across the lifespan, music strums our emotional strings. It's our first language and sometimes our last. For people suffering from dementia, the regions of the brain that store music memories are the last to deteriorate.[3] It's why people with Alzheimer's may be able to sing along to a favorite song from childhood but not remember the names of their caregivers.

In an interview with NPR, awe researcher Dacher Keltner said music allows us to feel "transcendent emotions" that can help counter the "epidemic of our times": loneliness. Keltner continued, "With music, we feel we're part of a community, and that has a direct effect on health and well-being."[4] Perhaps that's why music is central to many religions, rituals, and cultural traditions.

Take school concerts. At my kids' most recent spring concert, the music teacher opened the program by saying, "I often tell the kids to listen for 'goosebump moments'—moments where the harmony starts to come together and the voices blend. Tonight, I hope you have at least one goosebump moment."

For some parents, that may be when their child puffs out "Twinkle, Twinkle, Little Star" on the recorder with their third grade class. For others, it may be watching kindergartners, all dressed up, fidget their way through "This Land Is Your Land." For me, it was listening to the fourth grade handbell choir—the resonance of the bells paired with the kids' earnest precision had the audience in a hush. Making music together is a transformative, community-affirming ritual.

The Difference Between Noise and Sound (and Why It Matters)

Music has cascading benefits for children of all ages, supporting everything from literacy skills to emotional regulation. But before diving into music specifically, let's take a step back and look at our kids' sonic environments more holistically.

I'll start by introducing Nina Kraus, a neuroscientist and the director of Brainvolts, an auditory neuroscience laboratory housed at Northwestern University. When I picked up her book, *Of Sound Mind: How Our Brain Constructs a Meaningful Sonic World*, I expected a straightforward, scientific tome. What I found was a love letter to sound—wrapped up in rich research.

When I called Kraus to talk about her research, she agreed with that assessment. "It really is a love letter to how sound makes us who we are, and how sound connects us," she said. "We don't recognize it so well because it's intangible, but it's what's connecting you and me right now."

Kraus told me that sound is inextricably tied to our understanding of our world: "It has a huge impact on who we are and how we engage with the world." Because of that, Kraus wants parents to pay more attention to children's auditory environments.

All sounds—from background noise to music lessons—can influence brain development, she said. And because we live in a noisy world, not all sound is healthy—much less awe-inspiring. Some is just noise or, as Kraus defines it, "unwanted sound." We all know that very loud noises can damage our ears, but Kraus is also concerned about so-called "safe noise" and its effects on children. These constant, moderate amounts of noise that fill our lives "don't hurt our ears, but they hurt our brain." Think about when the dishwasher finishes its cycle or when the neighbor shuts off the leaf blower. "You hadn't even noticed that those sounds were there," said Kraus. "But when they are turned off, we breathe a sigh of relief."

Kraus says there's a reason we are more attuned to sounds at night too. From an evolutionary perspective, sound puts us on alert. Our ancestors needed to be able to detect threats in the darkness. This explains why I can sleep through my 6 a.m. alarm but jolt awake when I hear my kids' calls in the middle of the night. If you are the parent of a newborn, you likely notice this acutely. Noises—whether or not we are consciously aware of them—tax our brains because they keep us in a state of alertness. They set off our sensory smoke detector.

In high-noise environments, sound processing in the brain can become diminished, and there can also be increased neural noise, or as Kraus calls it, "background static in the brain." That's not great for kids' developing brains. So how do we shape a healthier sonic environment for our children and teens?

First, we need to pay more attention to the noises that fill their lives and consider which are unnecessary. For example, do you need a ping every time you get a notification on your phone or computer? Does that app your child is playing need the sound on to function, or are the beeps simply noise? As Kraus said, we are often guilty of being "too cavalier about the sounds that we salt and pepper our lives with."

Second, we can look for ways to reduce noise and tune in to nourishing sounds—such as those found in nature. "Noise is almost always human made, so listening to nature's music offers children and adults a rejuvenating auditory experience." Outdoor spaces, especially forests but even some city parks, are "teeming with sound," says Kraus. "There are brooks running, birds tweeting, and animals moving around in the thicket." These sounds help us connect to our environment and experience multisensory beauty.

Silence is also part of a healthy sonic diet. "We need a lot more wonder and silence in our lives. Quiet is part of sound. It's the space between the notes," says Kraus. Removing noisy distractions and stimuli allows our brains to relax and wander to new places. And that space can make room for awe.

"Last year, one of my friends was playing a beautiful song on the piano. I don't know what came over me, but I was so moved by this song that I knew I had to learn how to play it. So two friends took turns teaching me each part of that song. I had taken piano lessons from second to fifth grade, but I *hated* lessons and my parents eventually let me stop. And now, because of this moment, I have started to love piano again."—Celia, high schooler

Music and the Developing Brain

Noise can often detract from learning, but *music*—from beat-keeping to note-reading—can build cognitive skills. Even just listening to music can activate kids' cognitive, motor, reward, and sensory networks. "Music should be a part of every child's education," Kraus told me. "It should be a priority as important as learning to read and write."

Let's explore why. Take just one element of music: rhythm. Stop and think about what you instinctively did when your child fussed as a baby. You started to bounce or rock them, right? That rocking is rhythm—one of the core ingredients of music.

Early in Anita Collins's music education career, she noticed a connection between kids' ability to keep the beat in music class and their progress in literacy classes. Sometimes, she could bring an early reading issue to an administrator's attention simply from watching a five-year-old struggle to stay on beat. She began to wonder: *If we do more beat-keeping, could we have an impact on literacy skills?*

When I posed that question to Kraus, she responded with a resounding *yes*. "When we think about rhythm, we usually think about music. But there is rhythm in speech," said Kraus. "We use rhythm all the time for turn-taking, for emphasis. We know that the kids who have difficulty with rhythm skills—like following the beat or rhythm pattern—are also kids who tend to have difficulty with language skills, and this includes reading." Keeping a beat trains the brain to detect the sound patterns that are a key part of literacy. Even dancing around the house to music and banging on homemade drums can teach rhythm.

This research gets me thinking about the kids in my life. My son is driven by rhythm. He has been a bouncer from birth—never happier than when in a swing or on a trampoline. He still does some of his best thinking while bouncing on a yoga ball. When learning a new piano piece, he almost effortlessly grasps the timing and tempo of the music. Sitting still can be a challenge, but I can see all the benefits and beauty that have emerged from his body in motion.

I also think about all the times I, as an English teacher, clapped out poetry rhythms with middle schoolers. We beat-boxed Shakespeare and choreographed interpretive dances to Shel Silverstein. This clapping and moving helped some students grasp poetic meter for the first time. And I'm convinced that my own kids know their punctuation rules because they grew up hearing me "write" out loud, verbalizing commas, periods, and quotation marks as I sent myself voice texts while pushing them in a stroller or cooking dinner.

Here is another insight worth sharing: Musical skills are essentially a boot camp for executive function skills, including attention, memory, and task persistence. As Collins told me, "If we think about attention span as a muscle, we are strengthening that muscle every time we practice music. We learn one line, then we add a little bit more. One bar, then two bars, then the whole page."

But when it comes to music education, Kraus's vision is broader than cognitive acumen. It has something to do with our shared humanity. "Most kids are never going to be concert pianists. And that's not at all the goal. In this world, we need to be able to connect across languages and cultures. Through music, we can build bridges."

Music and Mental Health

If you walk into Alder Hey Children's Hospital in Liverpool, England, you might be greeted by birdsong. The hospital recorded the birds' sunrise concert at a local park, calling it "Wild Song at Dawn." Children can also listen to the birdsong as they receive injections or other treatments. The hospital told the BBC, "The children find it very calming, and it can help them de-stress before undergoing treatments or surgery."[5] Several studies have found that listening to birdsong can relieve anxiety and promote feelings of well-being.[6]

While few species can match birds for beauty, pitch, and rhythm, human-made music also has these same therapeutic benefits. In fact, music can be a robust mental health tool for tweens and teens to access on their own. They often curate playlists to match the mood and the moment or to help them process their feelings. Sharing playlists can be an act of connection and vulnerability—a way for people of any age to share a piece of who they are with friends and family. Hearing a song or artist that speaks to you can be mesmerizing.

Take the Swifties among us. In 2023, psychiatrist Suzanne Garfinkle-Crowell wrote a guest essay for *The New York Times* titled

"Taylor Swift Has Rocked My Psychiatric Practice." She explains that, for a subset of her patients, Taylor Swift has become a tool for expressing what might otherwise feel inexpressible. She writes, "'What would Taylor Swift do?' is a refrain among certain patients in my practice. Teenagers suffer for many reasons. One is being fragile and in formation—a human construction site. Another is being surrounded by others who are fragile and in formation. Ms. Swift articulates not only the treachery of bullying but also the cruelty just shy of it that is even more pervasive: meanness, exclusion, intermittent ghosting. She says: Borrow my strength; embrace your pain; make something beautiful with it—and then you can shake it off."[7]

Lisa Damour, psychologist and author of *The Emotional Lives of Teenagers,* is an expert in teenage anxieties. She wants parents and kids to know that some degree of stress and anxiety is not only normal but essential for human growth. "Somehow a misunderstanding has grown up about stress and anxiety where our culture now sees both as pathological," said Damour. "The upshot of that is that we have adults and young people who are stressed about being stressed and anxious about being anxious."

The teen years and stress go hand in hand—because change, even when positive, is stressful, and teenagers' lives are filled with change. Their bodies and brains are transforming, they usually switch schools at least once between grades 5 and 12, their academic workloads are increasing, and their social relationships are constantly evolving. The anxiety that comes with stretching to face these and other challenges is part of how humans develop strength, explained Damour.

When teens accept that some level of stress is inevitable and a sign of growth, they can spend less time worrying about stress and instead focus on their recovery tools. Damour told me that you can think about working through stress like a kind of exercise: "The good news is your mind recovers a lot faster than your muscles do. But you need to restore yourself so you can go right back in for another workout. Your job is to figure out how you like to recover. What's the system that really works for you?" Music, she said, is often at the top of the list for teens.

"I've always had a thing for music. When I was very young, I saw a DJ. I kept saying to my parents, *I want to do that.* So after a few years, they got me lessons. When I started to DJ, my passion grew. My ear for music helped me find the beats. Even before I started DJing, I could tell when there was going to be a new bar or a drop in the music before it happened—like instinct. Sometimes when I'm stressed or when my younger siblings are bickering, I go up to my room, listen to my favorite songs, and start scratching. When I'm DJing, I get lost in the moment."—Araya, age 12

How exactly does music work as a recovery tool? In a *Washington Post* essay, music therapist Raymond Leone wrote, "Music can have a profound effect on us. It can improve our physical and mental health by helping to reduce blood pressure, alleviate stress, and lead to a release of dopamine, a neurotransmitter that affects our mood and sense of happiness."[8]

Intrigued, I reached out to Leone, the medical music therapy director at A Place to Be, a therapeutic arts organization in Leesburg, Virginia. He told me that music is something we experience both physically and emotionally. "Our brains react to music differently than most anything else. When we hear or play music, multiple parts of our brains are active in both hemispheres," he said. "Music also creates emotion and prompts memories. When we hear a song that was prominent at an event in our lives—a wedding song, a breakup song, a parent's favorite song—it prompts our memories of the person or situation."

In other words, our lives have a soundtrack. Songs make and carry memories; music both evokes emotion and revives it. I could pair a song with almost every major event in my life. How about you? What song reminds you of your mom or dad or big brother or grandmother? What song still makes you tear up every time you hear it? If we experience awe while listening to a song at a concert, hearing that song on the radio puts us right back in touch with that feeling.

Using Music to Connect with Kids

During a recent workshop, I asked attendees to turn to someone else and share a song or music memory that gave them goosebumps. The audience was a mix of high schoolers and their teachers. The conversation was so animated that I let it go on for an extra five minutes. One teen got to hear about their teacher's first Grateful Dead concert. Another enjoyed telling a teacher why they listen to the *Dear Evan Hanson* cast recording on repeat.

The music that gives us goosebumps probably won't be *that song* for our kids. My father-in-law often insisted that my husband would learn to love opera by the time he was fifty. Nope, didn't happen. For our daughter's twelfth birthday, my husband made her a playlist with full liner notes of some of his favorite songs. Did she like every selection? No, but she loved the care that went into this gift. This last Christmas, she reciprocated, gifting her dad a playlist that merged her favorites from his album with additional songs that she thought they would both enjoy.

One of my son's favorite memories from first grade is "song share." Every Friday, his teacher invited two or three students to choose a favorite song to play for their classmates (prescreened for age appropriateness) and share why they like it—a fun twist on traditional show-and-tell. On the Friday drive home, he would recall each song and then ask me to play them again. He not only discovered new music, but he also strengthened his relationships with his classmates. Four years later, he will still say, "Alex is the one who introduced me to Alan Walker," or "I know this song! This was Max's song share!"

Given the emotions wrapped up in music, this is a great place to offer curiosity instead of judgment about kids' choices. Show an interest in what your kids are listening to. Be grateful if they let you glimpse their playlists. And make sure you get to blast your music, too, despite protests. Have a family dance party in the kitchen. Go check out a summer concert in the park. Sing loudly in the car. Find and share new artists that bring each family member joy.

My friend Tresa Edmunds knows that music can be a great medium for connecting with our kids. Edmunds is a writer and an activist who teaches self-care through the lens of disability, drawing on her wisdom as a "disabled parent of a disabled kid." Atticus is Edmunds's son. He was born prematurely and lives with multiple disabilities, including autism. Atticus is categorized as nonverbal. But as Edmunds told me, "He communicates all the time if you know how to listen."

She shared this reflection, "Atticus is fifteen now, and music has always been the language that connects us. Music is the bridge between his nonverbal autistic language and my spoken language. I think the power of music is that the body translates it before the brain does. The rhythm and the soundwaves of the instruments make it an embodied form of communication like no other method. With me and Atti, our language doesn't always make sense to each other. But we can both understand the meaning in the music."

Edmunds's words brought another story to my mind. In 2019, nine-year-old Ronan Mattin and his grandfather attended a concert by the Handel and Haydn Society (H+H). At the end of any orchestral performance, there is usually a pause after the music finishes and before the applause begins. Into the silence that followed the orchestra's performance of Mozart's "Masonic Funeral Music," Ronan's loud voice filled Boston's Symphony Hall: "WOW!"

The audience laughed and clapped. David Snead—the president and CEO of H+H—called it "one of the most wonderful moments I've experienced in the concert hall."[9] Audio of Ronan's exclamation went viral. And in 2024, poet Todd Boss and illustrator Rashin Kheiriyeh turned the moment into a picture book called *The Boy Who Said Wow*.

Here's something else to know about Ronan. Like Atticus, he is autistic and nonverbal. Before listening to that performance of Mozart, he had never said "wow" before. According to his family, he only spoke when "heavily prompted"—and only about wants and needs. This spontaneous vocalization gave thousands of people goosebumps because it communicated something ineffable, something that cannot be expressed in words. Five years after the "wow" moment, Snead told *The Boston Globe*, "It isn't often that you experience such a spontaneous, unfiltered expression of joy and awe as Ronan's 'Wow.' He said what everyone in the hall was feeling in that moment, but could not express— except Ronan, who just couldn't hold back. Maybe we need more of that in the concert hall."[10]

The Mandolin Solution: Aimee's Story

For Aimee Evans Hickman, music allowed her neurodivergent child to discover his authentic self. She shares their story in her own words and with her son's permission:

When my son, Leo, was eight years old, he wandered into the wrong room at school—only to discover a table full of classical mandolins. Finding himself alone with only his unyielding curiosity, he strummed his fingers across eight strings that sounded painfully out of tune to his persnickety ears. He picked up one of the bowl-backed instruments and began carefully turning pegs before the mandolin teacher, Ms. Laura, walked through the door.

Rather than scold him, she asked him to bring her the mandolin so that she could show him how it worked. She was astonished as she ticked down each string. He had tuned it perfectly by ear. Right then and there, Leo became Ms. Laura's mandolin student.

Ms. Laura's patience and enthusiasm were a gift to this neurodivergent boy, who was often challenged by his own restlessness. As a cello student at Baltimore School for the Arts, trying to sit still through hours of weekly orchestra rehearsals often left him feeling defeated. One day, he decided to bring his mandolin to school. In a moment of serendipity, that was the day Cuban/Venezuelan jazz pianist César Orozco was visiting the school. Leo found himself jamming with César.

This moment of musical improvisation transformed Leo's entire relationship with music. Three years later, after a derailing pandemic, Leo found himself attending a weekly jam session in the style of Django Reinhardt led by guitarist Michael Harris. This has cultivated his growth as a jazz mandolinist and has given him a nurturing, joyful community.

What began as a little boy wandering into the wrong room became a childhood and adolescence filled with music and mentors who guided Leo through some of life's biggest transitions. I've known ever since he touched his first mandolin that music would be a deep source of solace for him, but I didn't know it would also be the magic spell to forging his most rewarding relationships. Music gave him a sense of purpose and direction when the world seemed to bottom out. How grateful I am to every mentor who has improvised with Leo in music and in life.

The Importance of Sensory-Friendly Performances

There is one more piece of Ronan's story that stirs up a lot of emotion for me. After his *wow*—and before the public celebration of it—Ronan and his grandfather left a bit early so as not to "disturb" other patrons, as Ronan's grandfather worried might happen. I get it. Museums, plays, and concerts are not always friendly places for young children or for kids and teens with sensory needs. That can be a barrier to parents who want to expose their kids to these wonders but who worry about overstimulating their child and/or having their child be subjected to the judgment of others if they can't conform to rigid behavioral norms.

My kids' first large concert was the Wiggles—a children's band from Australia. The enormous auditorium exploded with pulsing music, squeals of delight, and small bodies squirming in the aisles. With each new song, the audience, including one of my kids, became more energized. Luckily, this was an environment that welcomed their calls, cheers, wiggles, and moves. But it was not an ideal environment for all kids. About halfway through the concert, my other child snuggled against me, ears covered to soften the din. As we drove home, the energized child wanted to listen to music the whole way home, but I kept the stereo off to allow the sibling time to recharge in peace.

Both of my kids enjoyed the concert, but they reacted differently to the sensory stimulation. Yes, my sound-sensitive child found a way to modulate the stimulus (and I envied the wisdom of the parents who had brought along noise-reducing headphones). But sensory overload can lead to emotional dysregulation for many kids. When that happens, an awesome experience can start to feel kind of awful.

My friend Becca's children recently acted in a community production in Flint, Michigan, that offered a designated "sensory-friendly performance"—a show that moderated lights, sounds, and transitions, among other things. When Becca asked her kids to reflect on this specific performance, the consensus was that "the burden on the performers was minimal, while the access and the joy for the audience was huge." Her nine-year-old noted, "It was not the hardest thing to change [the production]. I enjoyed it." Her seventeen-year-old added, "The sensory performance was a lot more laid back than I was expecting. I definitely think it's a worthwhile theater endeavor because we need options for more people to see cool stuff."

Sensory-friendly and family-friendly performances help ensure that auditory wonders are accessible to everyone. And thankfully, more and more performance groups and theaters are offering these shows. One of the leaders in this effort is Dan + Claudia Zanes, a children's music duo who make their shows "sensory friendly whenever possible (which has been most of the time)." They write:[11]

> When we say sensory friendly, we're indicating that all are welcome. Our goal is to create an environment that's as inclusive and accessible to everyone. The audience that has always felt comfortable and welcome at our shows is invited as well as people with diverse sensory needs.
>
> We've heard over and over from parents of children with disabilities that their child's responses in public spaces can lead to uncomfortable situations in which they feel judged or unwelcome. Sensory-friendly performances are a way of saying "come as you are, we're all in this together." We've seen firsthand how moving it can be when families who might not generally mix are able to enjoy music together. Once we experienced this, there was no turning back!

Reading their reflection brought tears to my eyes, because my family has experienced firsthand the care of Dan + Claudia Zanes. In the summer of 2017, our family moved across the country. In those first few weeks in our new home, my three-year-old struggled with the adjustment. On a particularly rough night, I opened my email to find Dan Zanes's newsletter. He was performing that weekend, only thirty minutes from our new home! Dan Zanes wasn't just any children's artist—he was my son's absolute FAVORITE.

6 Things to Look for in Sensory-Friendly Performances

If you're searching for sensory-friendly or family-friendly music experiences for your children, Dan + Claudia Zanes share six things to look for to ensure the experience is awe-some for kids:[12]

1. **Moderate Volume.** "We try to avoid jarring musical and sound transitions from soft to loud to soft again within the composition of the music."

2. **Moderate Lighting.** "House lights between 25 and 40, the elimination of strobe lights, and lighting focused on the audience are good ways to maintain a sensory-friendly environment."

3. **A Designated Quiet Alternative Area.** "If possible, beanbag chairs and a video monitor showing the action onstage are good for this area."

4. **A Visual Schedule.** "This can be as simple as an illustrated set list that lets families know what to expect next."

5. **Language to Indicate That All Are Welcome.** "Families with children who have disabilities often feel as though their child's behavior is being unfairly criticized. The purpose of a sensory-friendly show is to create an atmosphere that is welcoming to one and all."

6. **More Explicit Volunteer and Staff Training.** "This is often as simple as asking ushers and front-of-house personnel to be welcoming and to 'relax the rules' that might usually apply."

Misty-eyed, I clicked "reply," expressing my thanks for this well-timed concert. He wrote back within minutes, inviting my kid to meet him after the show.

The concert was held in a mid-sized room at a local hotel. Dan Zanes had just joined forces with Claudia. While the room was filled with children, the atmosphere was unexpectedly soothing. During the performance, Dan gave my son a shout-out by name and asked the audience to welcome him to Boston. My son beamed; he was filled with awe. The whole ride home, he kept repeating, "He's the bestest, bestest singer." The memory still makes me teary.

A Final Thought

I first met Emily Nelson when she was in my tenth grade English class. For one assignment, I asked students to turn a poem into a new art form—a painting, a sculpture, a dance, a song, a video. Emily quietly walked to the front of the room with her ukulele and sang an original song based on William Wordsworth's "The World Is Too Much with Us." When she finished, the room was silent. Mouth-agape silence. I had goosebumps. The students and I were collectively awestruck.

I caught up with Emily while writing this book. She is now a college senior majoring in music therapy, and she gets the last word for this chapter.

My earliest memories surrounding music were in church. I remember hearing a choir harmonize and feeling, "This is beautiful." I felt like I needed to be a part of it, so I'd sing the hymns at the top of my lungs. Hearing videos of me singing when I was four, I wasn't any good. But one day, an older man came up to me after church and said, "You are an inspiration. I just want you to know how much that touched me." I didn't understand it then, but I think a young child's voice in a beautiful place moved him.

As I got older, I developed stage fright for a while. Now that I'm in music school and performing all the time, I don't get that fear as often. But I have been surprised that some of my least "impressive" performances (on a technical level) have moved audiences the most because these songs moved me. The emotional content of the song is often more important to audiences than the melodic, rhythmic, or technical content.

I believe we communicate emotion through music. So much about emotion is hard to put into words, and yet music is such a great way to connect on that plane. I remember my first performance as part of a traveling 1940s USO-themed show in high school. A ninety-six-year-old World War II veteran lifted himself from his chair, tears streaming down his face. After the show, I decided to find him, shake his hand, and hear his story. As I talked to him, it was clear that what had evoked his emotion was not just the melody. It was that he felt seen.

Moments like these got me interested in music therapy. My group would sing at a senior center, and the staff would tell us, "This lady has not spoken for the past three days, and she's standing up. She's singing." Music does something to people on a spiritual level and a chemical level. It connects areas in the brain that aren't connected by regular speech.

Last semester, my practicum clinical placement was at a place that offers outreach and education to people experiencing homelessness. We provided music therapy classes. One technique we used was drumming. One person would start a rhythm, and then another person would add a rhythm. At the start, people would be hesitant. By the end, everyone was in this groove. Everyone's drumming hard, people are sweating, and they're all in. You could feel this collective movement from hesitation to confidence—and this sense of connection to everyone who was drumming with you. There's a lot of good research on that—how group drumming increases social connection to others and the ability to express oneself. But it's just wild that this happens without saying a single word.

Here's what I truly believe: Music will heal you, and it will heal the people around you.

5 Wonderful Ways to Enjoy Music with Kids

1. Tag the Emotion. Music can help build children's emotional literacy. Ask them to think about how different songs make them feel. Can they name a sad song? A happy song? A song that makes them want to dance? A song that relaxes their body?

2. List It. Many kids and teens love making playlists. Ask your kids to create family playlists for various occasions—like chore time, a family road trip, a birthday party, or a holiday dinner.

3. Feel the Beat. Clapping, stomping, and drumming to the beat are both fun for kids and good for their brain development. So turn on some music with a strong rhythm and get moving.

4. Make Instruments. Turn a food storage container and dry beans into a maraca. Loop different-sized rubber bands over a shoebox to make a guitar. Cut and tape together different lengths of straws to make a flute-pipe. Turn any container over to make a drum.

5. Find Music in the Community. There's nothing quite like experiencing live music, and once you start looking you will likely find plenty of it in your community: high school band and orchestra concerts, college a cappella groups, street-corner performers, concerts in the park or at a farmer's market, open mic night at a local coffee shop, church choirs. If you have little ones, many libraries have free music classes where kids can sing, dance, listen, and drum.

10 Awe-Inspiring Picture Books About Music

Music Is in Everything by Ziggy Marley and Ag Jatkowska. This colorful picture book shows kids that you can find music anywhere—in someone's laughter or even in the ocean waves. You don't need an instrument to hear beautiful sounds; you just need to listen to the world around you.

Because by Mo Willems and Amber Ren. *Because* tells the story of a young girl's journey to becoming a composer. Through whimsical illustrations, we watch our protagonist fall in love with music and take the stage.

Wild Symphony by Dan Brown and Susan Batori. Follow along with Maestro Mouse on a musical journey! Kids will see animals of all different kinds—from blue whales to tiny beetles, each with their own special secret. Parents and children can scan over each page with a free smartphone app to play a different song.

Never Play Music Right Next to the Zoo by John Lithgow and Leeza Hernandez. A concert turns chaotic when the animals break out of the zoo! The animals stomp across the stage and begin to play the instruments themselves. Based on one of John Lithgow's most famous melodies, this book contains a CD of John and an orchestra playing the song (or you can look it up online).

Listen: How Evelyn Glennie, a Deaf Girl, Changed Percussion by Shannon Stocker and Devon Holzwarth. This picture book biography tells the inspirational story of drummer Evelyn Glennie. Evelyn's early passion for music was nearly shattered when she began to lose her hearing at age eight. But she learned that she could feel the musical vibrations in her body and has toured the world as a professional solo-percussionist.

Dancing Hands: How Teresa Carreño Played the Piano for President Lincoln **by Margarita Engle and Rafael López.** Young piano virtuoso Teresa Carreño fled fighting in her home country of Venezuela to come to the United States just as the Civil War was breaking out. As her fame grew, eight-year-old Teresa was personally invited by President Lincoln to play for him at the White House shortly after he signed the Emancipation Proclamation.

Sing a Song: How "Lift Every Voice and Sing" Inspired Generations **by Kelly Starling Lyons and Keith Mallett.** Using the Black National Anthem as framing and inspiration, this book looks at Black history since 1900 through five generations of one family.

The Girl Who Heard the Music: How One Pianist and 85,000 Bottles and Cans Brought New Hope to an Island **by Marni Fogelson, Mahani Teave, and Marta Álvarez Miguéns.** Born on Easter Island, a girl named Mahani learned to play on her small island's only piano. After touring the world as a concert pianist, Mahani returned home and built a music school out of recycled ocean trash that was plaguing her home. This book is based on her true story.

Every Little Thing **by Cedella Marley and Vanessa Brantley-Newton.** Adapting the lyrics to her father Bob Marley's beloved song "Three Little Birds," Cedella Marley reimagines them as telling the story of a young child's ups and downs.

The Boy Who Said Wow **by Todd Boss and Rashin Kheiriyeh.** This book is based on the true story of a boy who was so transfixed by an orchestra performance that he uttered a loud "wow" that was heard around the musical world!

CHAPTER THREE

THE WONDER OF ART

That's what I'm interested in: the space in between, the moment of imagining what is possible and yet not knowing what that is.
—*Julie Mehretu*

"Find your muse." That was the assignment I gave my seventh grade English class as we walked into the Metropolitan Museum of Art in New York City.

We had been reading ekphrastic poetry in our New Jersey classroom, and this was the culminating activity. *Ekphrasis*, which means "description" in Greek, is a poetic translation of visual art. Basically, a writer takes a piece of art and uses it to inspire a poem. Think of Keats's "Ode on a Grecian Urn" (based on Greek pottery) or Anne Sexton's "The Starry Night" (based on Van Gogh's painting of the same name). Contemporary poets have also found this form appealing—like Asiya Wadud's "Shorn, treaded red," based on the painting *Satellites 27* by Etel Adnan.

Sure, I could have projected a piece of art in the classroom and asked my students to write a poem. But the history teacher was planning a museum trip *anyway*, so I bartered for a bit of time.

On the bus, I handed each student a paper with these instructions:

1. When you arrive at the museum, you will have one hour to immerse yourself in a piece of art.

2. Survey all your choices. Find a piece of art that speaks to you for any reason, a piece you want to explore. Write everything you see in detail—perhaps even sketch it. Note angles, colors, shapes, patterns.

3. Notice your reaction. What does this piece make you think about or feel? What questions do you have? (*Why is she carrying the apple? What is he looking at in the distance? Why is the sky painted green?*) Jot down words or phrases that you might include in a poem.

It's impressive how far choice goes with kids. My students scattered about in five interlocking galleries—some settling in the European sculpture room with others heading to modern or contemporary galleries. I watched a student who had been resistant to our poetry unit sit at the foot of Jean-Antoine Houdon's sculpture *Winter*, scribbling away in her notebook. The bronze woman clothed in a thin scarf seems to shiver with cold. Another sat with Georgia O'Keeffe's *Black Abstraction*, staring at the rolling hills of darkness punctuated by a tiny bright circle resting in the painting's center.

This field trip was on my mind when, years later, I took my children to the Museum of Fine Arts, Boston, for the first time. They were ten and seven, and the size of the museum made it impossible to see everything in a day. So I picked a few galleries and gave them a challenge: Find one piece of art you would take home with you if you could. Each time we entered a new room, the kids scrambled about, looking for a piece that spoke to them. I did the same. Once we had found our favorites, we traveled to each other's choices. I remember my son's bubbling excitement when he showed us Thomas Cole's dramatic landscape *Expulsion from the Garden of Eden*—the exploding volcano! The violent winds! The jagged rocks! And the *teeny-tiny* Adam and Eve entering the world. His sister was drawn to modern and contemporary art, to pieces that provoked more questions than answers. Seeing their reactions—both to what they loved and what they didn't—was fascinating and reminded me that there is so much about my kids' internal worlds that I'm still discovering.

Art evokes awe: making art, seeing art, and even noticing visual design elements in the world at large, from a seashell's Fibonacci spiral to a snowflake's hexagonal structure. And it turns out that there is rich research on how art supports our children's cognitive growth and overall well-being.

How Art Benefits Kids

It's old news that art classes are often the first to go when school budgets get tight, particularly in underresourced districts serving students in low socioeconomic communities. In 2013, nearly 30 percent of schools in Houston, Texas, had no fine arts teachers. Houston's art community and some philanthropic donors rallied together to offer art education programs to schools. When more schools applied for funding than could be accommodated, researchers found an opportunity to conduct a large-scale experiment. Would there be contrasting outcomes between kids who were exposed to art and those who were not?

Researchers gathered data at twenty-one schools that received arts education (roughly eight thousand students in grades 3 through 8). They then compared the results to twenty-one schools that did not receive extra arts programming. As education reporter Jill Barshay wrote, "The students in both groups were demographically similar: One quarter of the students were Black, two-thirds were Hispanic. More than 85 percent of their families were poor enough to qualify for free or reduced-price lunch. Of course, it wasn't a blind test. The students knew they were getting art and there was no placebo, but it's as close as you get to a pharmaceutical drug trial in education."[1]

The schools that received funding were visited by teaching artists and went on field trips to museums and music events. It was a bit of an "artistic potpourri," as Barshay describes it—not an established, systematized curriculum. But after one year, the results started coming in, including these:[2]

| The arts-funded schools saw improvements in student behavior and students' social and emotional skills—including an increase in empathy and compassion.

| These same students were more engaged in their learning and reported more college-related aspirations.

| On Texas standardized tests, students who were exposed to art got higher marks on writing.

After this short exposure to art, students did not have higher standardized math scores than their peers. However—and this is important—they did not experience a *drop* in math scores. Policymakers often argue that time spent in arts classes will detract from learning the core subjects. This did not turn out to be the case.

Art and Spatial Reasoning

The Houston study is just a piece of the story when it comes to how art helps kids flourish. There is some evidence that becoming proficient in art changes the very structure of the brain. For example, a study examining brain scans of visual arts students revealed that they have more neural matter in areas relating to fine-motor movements and visual imagery than their non-art-school peers.[3] Rebecca Chamberlain, one of the researchers, told the BBC that "people who are better at drawing really seem to have more developed structures in regions of the brain that control for fine motor performance and what we call procedural memory."[4] This brain region is also linked to creativity and spatial skills—including the ability to manipulate visual images in your head, combining and deconstructing them.

The words *spatial skills* in this study caught my attention. A few years ago, I published a series of articles on kids and spatial reasoning. This topic doesn't get much attention in parenting forums, and you don't find many viral articles on it. But the more I have learned, the more I want to share the research with parents. Here's the essential takeaway: There's a robust link between spatial reasoning and academic achievement in math, science, and the arts.

In my research, I came across the work of engineering professor Sheryl Sorby. She was troubled by how many students—and particularly young women—dropped out of engineering programs after their first year. She had a hypothesis: The first engineering courses at most colleges are highly spatial. Discouraged by struggles in the introductory courses and believing they weren't cut out for the program, some students simply changed majors. "A lot of people believe that spatial intelligence is a fixed quantity—that you either have good spatial skills or you don't—but that's simply not true," Sorby told me. This misperception is particularly harmful to young women. Sorby noted that, in general, young girls are less likely to be encouraged to play with toys that strengthen spatial intelligence. Case in point: When my daughter was born in 2011, Target still had literal "Blue" and "Pink" toy aisles. Guess where all the blocks, marble runs, Legos, car tracks, and other building toys were located? The Blue Zone. Target finally ended color-coding in 2015, but if you type "toys for boys" and "toys for girls" into the search bar on Amazon, you'll find a digital version of these aisles.

But there's good news: Spatial skills can be taught. So Sorby developed a "short introduction to spatial visualization" class to support incoming engineering students. What did this class include? A lot of art.

Sorby taught students how to sketch figures from multiple perspectives, look at cross-sections of objects, and create 3-D objects through paper-folding exercises. Students who took the class strengthened their spatial skills, improved their grades in all their

STEM classes, and were more likely to graduate with an engineering degree.[5]

Awe-inspiring, right? It's also a great reminder that artists use math. Musicians use science. Engineers draw and write. Naturalists paint. Dancers know a lot about physiology. One teenager I know participated in a six-week art internship at the James Webb Space Telescope Mission Operations Center. Not a science internship—an *art* internship. For his final project, he composed a song using the sonification of light from a binary star system as the foundational tone and rhythm. He then overlaid it with ambient electric guitar and electric mandolin. Finally, he set the whole thing to an abstract animation that explored the awe that comes from sitting with the overwhelming vastness of space.

As I write this paragraph, one of my children is working on a science project about the "physics of drawing" and the other is sketching made-up hybridized animals—like a mix between a wolverine and a Tasmanian tiger—while chatting with me about cloning research. Are these artistic or scientific projects? Yes and yes.

Art and Mental Health

When our kids need to express their emotions, they communicate through behavior, through play, and through words. They also communicate through art. As James S. Gordon says, as shared in the book *Your Brain on Art: How the Arts Transform Us* by Susan Magsamen and Ivy Ross, "In my experience, art goes beyond words in helping us to understand what's going on with ourselves and to understand what we should do with it."[6]

This quote makes me think about a former colleague of mine who lost her husband at a young age. At the time, she had two children under age ten, and she made it a priority to find therapeutic support for them. She was surprised to find that most of those counseling sessions included art. She described how one of her children covered their paper in intense markings that looked like anger exploding. The other drew intricate pictures of herself with her dad, pulling from her memories. For both, she said, art offered a noticeable relief and opened channels of communication.

My friend's experience echoes findings on art's mental and emotional benefits. After reviewing twenty years of studies, researchers Heather L. Stuckey and Jeremy Nobel found that making art has many positive effects:[7]

| It helps people express experiences that are "too difficult to put into words."

| It offers a cathartic release of, and a refuge from, intense emotions.

| It provides creative ways to express grief and pain.

| It facilitates verbal communication of thoughts and feelings.

| It reduces cortisol related to stress.

| It decreases anxiety and increases positive emotions.

These findings are true across the lifespan: A study in Britain found that adults who made art at least once a week were more content with their lives than those who did not.[8] A longitudinal study out of Japan found that people who regularly crafted or painted had less cognitive impairment later in life.[9]

Art even benefits our youngest, most vulnerable kids. One team of researchers wanted to investigate whether arts education could attenuate the effects of poverty. Could art "get under the skin" and reduce cortisol levels for economically disadvantaged preschoolers?

The researchers studied 310 three- to five-year-old children at a Head Start school in Seattle, Washington. Students received visual arts, music, and dance classes in addition to their regular curriculum. The researchers swabbed the children's cheeks at different points in the day to measure hormone levels—particularly cortisol, sometimes known as the "stress hormone." Here is what they found: When children participated in an arts class, they had lower cortisol levels than when they had participated in a regular homeroom class at the same time of day. On days when kids had more than one arts class, their cortisol was lower than on days when they had fewer arts classes.[10]

Here's why this research is important: Poverty leaves biological markers in children, including elevated stress hormones and inflammation. There is evidence that toxic stress of any kind—loss, abuse, community violence—can affect the structure of the developing brain, leading to struggles with learning, self-regulation, and physical and mental health.[11] So whether your kids are experiencing significant challenges or those inevitable smaller struggles, art is one additional resource you can employ to support them.

Unleashing Kids' Inner Artists

As a parent, I have felt awe in seeing the art my kids produce—not for its precision, but for what it reveals to me about their inner selves and how their minds work.

When my son was struggling with worries about creatures in the closet, he drew a "Book of Monsters." Page after page of scribbled fiends, each with a very silly name. Did my kid do this consciously? All I know is that I didn't suggest this art activity. He came up with this strategy for combatting mental monsters all on his own. I also think of the hours he has spent designing intricate logos for dozens of imaginary sports teams, drawing detailed maps of imaginary countries, crafting new alphabets, and making symmetrical designs.

These days, my daughter fills sketchbook after sketchbook with art, no longer sharing as many of the pictures with me. But then again, I was a journal keeper as a tween. I understand how personal those notebook pages can be, whether they contain images or words, so I respect this need for privacy while quietly cheering on this new passion.

Feeling Seen by Art: Susanna's Story

My friend Susanna Driscoll, a physician by training, has spent the last two years in and out of the hospital for a different reason: Her young daughter has cancer. One day, she shared with me about how she found the hospital's corridor of art—and what it means to her. Here's how she tells it.

My daughter has had a prolonged hospitalization for cancer treatment. On her good days, when we both feel as if we're going stir-crazy in the hospital room, we leave the oncology ward and walk up and down the hospital corridors. At first, I just wanted to move, but I discovered the hospital displayed a number of art exhibits, most from local artists, and I found myself wanting to see the pieces again and again.

The appeal of some pieces was obvious, because they were beautiful, bright, and sunny. Who wouldn't appreciate a view like that during a Wisconsin February? But I also felt drawn to the dark and tumultuous works. They whispered to the reality and validity of my anger, fear, and confusion. One artist made a series of works using thin wire and fragile twigs arranged in different shapes in shadow boxes. They looked like they would break apart if someone slammed a door too hard, but there they were, intact for the moment, like my sanity.

I don't know when I have ever appreciated art as much as I have appreciated it during my daughter's prolonged illness. I've found both escape from the difficulty of my current reality and also mirror-like representations of the thoughts and feelings I've had in it. There is a feeling of community, of not being alone, of resonating with the common and complex experience of being human, and that is something I need right now.

Perhaps your kid has a natural inclination toward the visual arts or maybe they need a little encouragement. Whichever way they lean right now, encouraging them to engage with art has benefits. To understand more about how to do that, I contacted Louisa Penfold, the co-chair of Arts and Learning at the Harvard Graduate School of Education.

Penfold described visual art as a "language that allows children to communicate in ways that can't always be done through words and numbers." Our education system focuses heavily on literacy and numeracy—words and numbers. "And both of those things are very important," Penfold told me. "But not everything in the world can be communicated through those two modes." Art is a multimodal way to engage with the world and "an inquiry into the unknown." Penfold said that art prompts kids to ask better questions, think creatively, and employ critical thinking—all of which are key to children's learning and development. The arts also cultivate ways of thinking about the world from multiple perspectives, helping kids and teens understand that there are many ways of being in it. "The arts are a human right for kids," said Penfold. "When the arts get marginalized, that has major implications for children's holistic learning and development."

"When I'm making art, I'm happy. I especially love drawing cats. Lately, I've been realizing that when I'm drawing a cat with its mouth open, or hissing, I do the same action. I guess it's easier to draw an expression if I'm making the one I'm trying to draw. I draw every day, usually for hours. When my pencil touches the paper, it's magic. My worries just melt away. Everybody has a hobby they love. For me, drawing is my passion, my wonder, my happy place. It is what I love."—Paige, age 13

In our homes, she said, parents can think more intentionally about creating artistic experiences for children. Art directly taps into the definition of awe: "what we feel when we encounter something vast, wondrous, or beyond our ordinary frame of reference."[12] Artists often talk about feeling a "gravitational pull toward the unknown," said Penfold. It might be a sudden insight, goosebumps, or an urgency to create something: to build, to sculpt, to put pen to paper, to whoosh paint over a canvas. Art is a way to explore the unknown within and outside us.

"You can see that process manifesting with children as well," Penfold told me. "They'll have a curiosity about something, and that is the starting point for them to create an artwork." These moments of inspiration are fulfilling and unpredictable—another reason to become an everyday awe-seeker. "I think this feeling motivates people on the weekends to be like, *I'm going to go and see this art show*, or *There's this random performance happening down at the local park. Let's go.*"

Penfold also has some practical advice for parents as they seek to unleash kids' inner artists.

| Curate your space. Have age-appropriate art-making tools readily accessible: scissors, paint, construction paper, crayons, glue, and so on. Expose your kids to various art styles, including work that is culturally relevant to your family.

| Aim for the sweet spot. Sometimes adults introduce artists or new techniques in a didactic way—with a specific drawing to reproduce or craft to create. Other adults may say, "Oh, I'm just going to put a bunch of materials out and let the kids do whatever." Both have their place. But the sweet spot is giving kids freedom for creative experimentation while offering some structure or asking them questions that inspire them, push their creative thinking, or increase their skills.

⏐ Foster artistic play. Letting young children play with various materials can help spur their imaginations. For example, put out cardboard and items from recycling and let kids explore. Add some clothespins or tape and see how they use that with the items. After they play and build, show them pictures of works by artists like Louise Nevelson and see if that spurs more ideas for how to combine the objects. Allow kids to turn non-art materials into artistic tools—like using kitchen utensils to make shadow puppets or using acorns and sticks to build a fairy house.

Not everyone is eager to jump into artmaking. Parents might feel reticent, and we can unconsciously communicate that to our kids. Have you ever said in front of your child "I'm terrible at drawing" or "I'm just not artistic"?

"People's understanding of art is based on the opportunities they've had in their own life," said Penfold, "and how art has been taught in schools is not always about cultivating creativity and playfulness. Sometimes, it's very much [about] right and wrong." So if hearing that kids should be making art and playing with materials in an open-ended way is new to you, you're not alone.

To encourage your kids' creativity, start simple. Offer art materials and let them play. Over time, introduce new tools or show them a painting, sculpture, or piece of pottery that you like. Think about your children's interests and how those might intersect with art. As Penfold told me, "When you think about the process that professional artists engage with, the creation of large-scale artworks always begins with small-scale experimentation. That is the philosophy parents need to remember: that your efforts can be small-scale and profoundly affect children's learning and development."

My sibling Ray Farmer is an artist and art educator. When we were chatting by phone the other day, Ray shared one of their favorite memories from working at the Chicago Children's Museum: "For one of our early childhood workshops, we got out a bunch of cardboard boxes, paint, sponges, and tape for the two- to five-year-olds—with the loose prompt to transform these boxes into a city. The kids were entranced, like, *Oh my goodness! Look at what I can do with all this!*"

You don't always need special art tools, Ray told me, because your home and neighborhood are already filled with materials. Take something ordinary in your life and transform it. Ray offered these ideas: "Let your kids use blankets and furniture to turn the family room into a magical new place with comfy hideaways. Or use colored tape to decorate the kitchen table with patterns and designs. If you find some sticks and acorns in the park, ask, *What could we turn this into?* Art is all about being curious and playful. The ordinary becomes a little more extraordinary." When you allow kids to experiment with art, they are often "really surprised by their own imaginations," said Ray, "and I feel like there is a lot of awe in that."

Until Ray shared this, I had never really thought about decorating as an awe-inspiring art activity. Yet my kids still talk about the babysitter who let them build a blanket-and-pillow fort. They don't remember her name, but they remember eating Goldfish crackers and listening to the *Mary Poppins* soundtrack inside the quilted walls. They also reminisce about the "Comfytown" they built with a cousin, using every blanket, pillow, and stuffed animal in the house. My kids start planning Halloween decorations in September and begin cutting out snowflakes for the windows in November. For years, Ray traveled in to help us hang Christmas-tree lights, but these last two years my son has taken over the job, telling me, "Ray taught me how to do this. I know the process for getting it to look just right." When the tree is finally lit and the house lights dimmed, we collectively admire the sparkling branches in hushed delight.

Being an Awesome Art Critic

It's easy to dole out general praise when your kid holds up a picture for you to admire: *Nice! Great job! I love it!* But watch how their face lights up when you offer more specific feedback—observations about their creativity and effort. Here's what that might sound like:

- "I see swirls in the sky! It looks like it's a windy day."
- "You used four different colors in that flower. It looks so happy and friendly."
- "You put so many animals in your jungle. You must have spent a long time working on this."
- "There's so much expression in this person's face. You really captured their emotion."

You can also engage with your kids about their art. Louisa Penfold shares these five questions you can ask:

1. What would you like me to notice first about your creation?
2. Can you tell me about the trickiest part of making this?
3. What were you feeling when you made this artwork?
4. Can you tell me why you chose those colors/shapes/materials?
5. What would you do differently if you were to make this artwork again?

Let's Go See Some Art

I had barely turned seventeen when I left my home in Utah and boarded a plane by myself to Boston to start college at Boston University. I had only been east of Denver once. While Boston is small compared to New York City or Los Angeles, it was the grandest place I'd ever seen. Wandering the city those first few days made me feel small in the best of ways.

My introductory education class that very first semester was an unexpected experience. The professor, Steve Tigner, never used the word *awe*, but looking back now, I can see how every assignment, every reading, and every discussion seemed designed to evoke this emotion. He wanted us to reframe how we saw the task of teaching. We read poetry. We studied philosophy. We explored really big questions. We wrote and wrote and wrote. And once a week, we went on a field trip to see art. A gallery in the Museum of Fine Arts, Boston. The steps of the Boston Public Library. And the Isabella Stewart Gardner Museum.

Gardner was an art collector, and she designed her home to be a museum, living in private quarters on the fourth floor. She installed the paintings, murals, and furniture to create a sense of intimacy for patrons wandering through bedrooms and sitting rooms. The grand jewel of the museum is the four-story atrium in the center, teeming with plants and flooded with light from the glass ceiling. I spent the entire field trip with my mouth agape. I had never seen a building like this.

I began using the atrium as a favorite study space, often walking the mile from my dorm to the museum. Being surrounded by art, light, and plants gave me a sense of "small self" that comes with awe—but in a different way than staring up at the downtown skyscrapers. Two years later, I was reading in the museum when Dr. Tigner brought in a new group of freshmen. He took a picture of me leaning against a marble column, absorbed in a novel, and framed it as a gift. I hung it in my classroom for years. That picture reminded me that a singular experience with awe—in my case, a field trip to an art museum—can have unexpected ripple effects for years to come.

Last year, I took my daughter to the Isabella Stewart Gardner Museum for the first time. It felt almost sacred, and I was nervous with anticipation. Her mouth, like mine, dropped open with a *wow* when she saw the flourishing atrium. I don't know if she will experience ripple effects from that day, but I'll keep seeking experiences like these on my kids' behalf.

With all that said, I know that going to art museums isn't at the top of everybody's favorite-things list. Perhaps you were dragged through one as a child until your feet ached. Maybe you had an underwhelming reaction to art you were "supposed" to like. If you are willing to give art museums another chance, keep reading to listen in on my conversation with Queena Ko, the director of education at the Noguchi Museum in New York.

Designed by the Japanese American sculptor Isamu Noguchi, this was the first museum to be created by a living artist to showcase their own work. Ko told me, "I think the Noguchi Museum is a particularly aligned place for inspiring awe because the museum itself was established by an artist. The space was designed to facilitate a particular way of encountering work, walking around work, and living with work. During his lifetime, [Noguchi] really encouraged visitors to touch and sit on and play with his sculptures. You can feel that when you're in this space."

In Ko's experience, kids often respond to art with more awe than adult visitors do. Adults often have "preconceived notions about museums and expectations of propriety," she said. Take a sculpture called *Magic Ring*—essentially a large stone circle. Noguchi described it as a ring drawn in the sand by Merlin. That description and a quick glance are enough for some patrons. But kids often walk around the circle, jump inside it, sit with it, and come up with alternate ideas about its purpose—such as being a portal to another dimension.

The point of taking kids to see art is not simply to impart knowledge about art history. It's about allowing them to have a conversation with art. Skilled museum educators use an "inquiry-first" approach, said Ko. That's a practice that we can adopt as parents.

Inquiry requires you to slow down. Observe a piece closely, notice your responses (without judging them), ask questions, wonder *why* and *what if*. As Ko told me, "Questioning is truly at the core of artmaking." For example, try asking your kids, "If you could talk to this artist, what would you ask them?" Ko's words remind me of Harvard's Project Zero "See, Think, Wonder" thinking routine, which can be adapted for art inquiry:[13]

- What do you see?
- What does it remind you of?
- What does it make you wonder?

Museums and art classes are prominent places to find and create art. But art is everywhere once you start to pay attention. Public spaces have statues and sculptures. Beautiful buildings—old and new—can inspire us. Bridges are artistic and engineering feats. Farmer's markets feature stalls from local artists. Cities have street art and murals. Many places of worship contain purposeful art and design elements. And, of course, libraries have books. And I'm not just talking about books about artists; picture books are a wonderland of accessible art.

A Final Thought

When I reread notes from my interviews while writing this chapter, I was struck by how often teaching artists used the words *unknown* and *uncertainty* to describe the experience of seeing and making art. Most of us are not comfortable with uncertainty. We don't like waiting to hear if we got the job or what the test results say. And as parents, we *especially* don't like not knowing for certain that our kids will be okay, right-now-and-forever-thank-you.

These reflections remind me of a pair of conversations I had a few years ago that I still think about. First, a parent of a high school sophomore said to me, "I'm just so worried that my daughter doesn't seem to have a clue what she wants to do professionally. College is right around the corner, and she needs to figure it out soon!" Later that very day, a high school junior came into my office to vent: "Why does everyone keep asking me what I want to do with my life?! I'm seventeen! Right now, I'm just trying to *live* my life—and get some sleep, which is hard to do with all the homework and activities I have."

Natalie Potts, the visual arts department chair at Shady Side Academy, a private preK–12 school in Pittsburgh, knows how much pressure teens are under. I met Potts at a Challenge Success conference, which brought together parents, students, and educators to explore how we can help broaden our definition of "successful." Potts has long been interested in the intersection of art and awe, and she has shaped her art room to be a place where teens can play, wonder, and "leave space for *not* knowing."

"Leave space for not knowing." Let's sit with those five words for a while. Essentially, that stressed-out high school junior who came to my office was pleading, *Can't I just have some space to live in the uncertainty of growing up and figuring myself out? Do I have to plan out the rest of my life right now?* Potts explained that "looking for uncertainty and spending time deliberately not knowing are not typically celebrated in school." But art allows kids to embrace "not knowing" in a way that is "low stakes, fun, and unexpected." When we make art, says Potts, we get to "play with ideas without having to provide answers to questions as a condition of successful work." Potts draws inspiration from a mentor who told her, "Artists have special freedom to be wrong because we're not about being right."

Kids are wired for wonder—they are eager to explore the world and figure out how things work. They ask a lot of questions. But as they get older, many become increasingly concerned about getting the *right* answer, studying the *right* material for the test, and taking the *right* classes to position themselves for the *right* colleges. What if the awe that comes from nature, music, and art were able to fuel a more robust concept of success? What if it allowed us to ask better questions and find more meaningful answers?

That's the topic we'll tackle next.

5 Wonderful Ways to Make and View Art with Kids

1. Head Outside. Go outside with a notebook. Draw some of the shapes you see in nature (a leaf, a spider web, a piece of grass). Use chenille stems to turn one of those shapes into a three-dimensional sculpture. Take a walk around your neighborhood with your kids. What shapes do you see? When you return home, draw or paint a picture of some of the shapes you saw on your walk.

2. Beautiful Oops. Read Barney Saltzberg's *Beautiful Oops!* together. Drop some paint on a piece of paper or take an old drawing that you "messed up" and turn it into something new and beautiful. Here's a variation on that: Cut out a portion of someone else's art or photography (from a printout or magazine), glue it on to a piece of paper, and then make it your own! Perhaps one of Van Gogh's butterflies ends up on a T. rex's hat.

3. Chalk It Up. Sidewalk chalk invites exploration. Compared to a piece of paper, a driveway or sidewalk is an enormous canvas! And drawing with chalk is a full-body experience. Try creating a mural, drawing inspiring messages for the community, or designing a sprawling hopscotch court, with all the numbers (and letters too).

4. Family Art Time. Place some art supplies onto the kitchen table, put on some music, and have some family art time. Let your kids see you experimenting and having creative fun alongside them (and leave the self-deprecating comments unsaid!).

5. Read Picture Books. Some of my favorite artists are picture book illustrators. When you read picture books with your kids, you can read both the words and the pictures, exploring the details that add dimension to the story. Even tweens and teens love the nostalgia that comes from rereading old favorites (and being read to).

10 Awe-Inspiring Picture Books About Art

Anna at the Art Museum **by Hazel Hutchins, Gail Herbert, and Lil Crump.** Anna's first trip to the museum isn't going well. Everything seems boring and there are so many rules for an energetic kid. But when a guard lets her enter an off-limits art restoration section, she begins to look at the art in a new way.

This Art Is for the Birds **by Susan Bednarski.** An artistic New York City pigeon thinks his paintings belong in a museum, and he and his friends set out to make this dream come true. The book contains delightfully "pigeonized" versions of famous art.

The Noisy Paint Box: The Colors and Sounds of Kandinsky's Abstract Art **by Barb Rosenstock and Mary GrandPré.** Vasya Kandinsky was a groundbreaking abstract artist who heard colors as sounds and saw sounds as colors. This book is a celebration of his life and art, as well as an introduction to synesthesia.

Maybe Something Beautiful: How Art Transformed a Neighborhood **by F. Isabel Campoy, Theresa Howell, and Rafael López.** This lovely book is based on the true story of San Diego's Urban Art Trail. In a drab urban landscape, people of all ages came together to make vibrant public art.

When I Draw a Panda **by Amy June Bates.** The narrator is a young girl who loves to draw—but doesn't love that her circles come out "wonky." When a panda she draws comes to life, it teaches her a little something about embracing her playfulness and creativity.

How to Make a Bird **by Meg McKinlay and Matt Ottley.** Perfect for artists of any age, this book is all about being a creator and how it feels to put your creations into the world.

Radiant Child: The Story of Young Artist Jean-Michel Basquiat **by Javaka Steptoe.** In this nonfiction picture book biography of the famed Haitian-American artist Basquiat, Steptoe replicates the vibrant style and feel of his work.

Harold and the Purple Crayon **by Crockett Johnson.** Written in 1955, this book tells the story of a four-year-old whose magic crayon leads him on an unforgettable adventure. He discovers he has the power to create a new world through his art.

Yayoi Kusama: From Here to Infinity **by Sarah Suzuki and Ellen Weinstein.** Have you seen the iconic dots of Japanese artist Kusama? If not, this book is a great introduction to one of the world's most heralded contemporary artists.

Sonia Delaunay: A Life of Color **by Cara Manes and Fatinha Ramos.** Based on the life and art of Delaunay—an artist and fashion designer in the early 1900s—this book follows Delaunay and her young son as they take a trip into one of her paintings. He learns more about how his mother sees the world through the lens of color and shape.

CHAPTER FOUR

THE WONDER OF BIG QUESTIONS

I am just a child that has never grown up. I still keep asking these how and why questions. Occasionally, I find an answer.
—Stephen Hawking

One night when my son was six, he called me to his bedroom at nearly 11 p.m. "Mommy! I need to know: What is past the universe? If you fly out of the universe, where are you? Also, I need a drink." Just last week, my kids spent the car ride home discussing the question *Does time exist, or is it something humans invented?* This led to further questions, such as *Is there such a thing as the present if the present instantly becomes past?* Eventually, my daughter said, "When I think about time too much, it feels like my head will explode!" These are Big Questions.

When these same kids were preschoolers, they asked *why* questions so often that I started to write them down. These are a handful of their queries:

- Why can't I drink water and breathe at the same time?

- Why do slugs make slime?

- Why are they called hot dogs if they aren't made from dogs?

- Why don't dande*lions* roar?

- Why are they called summer salts (i.e., somersaults) instead of winter peppers?

Later, these questions became fodder for my picture book *You Wonder All the Time*. When, recently, I read this book to a group of kindergartners in New Jersey, they generated dozens of their own wonderful questions, like *Why do I get dizzy when I spin around? Why do lemons have to be so sour? Why does the earth move but we don't feel it? How do people grow?*

Here's an unsurprising factoid: The average four-year-old asks approximately seventy questions each day.[1] If you are currently raising a preschooler, that number may feel low. But think of it this way: Childhood is a barrage of "firsts." First step. First time tasting a lemon. First snowstorm. First time walking into school. These firsts slow down the older we get, so adults sometimes forget what it is like to see, hear, or experience something for the first time. But it's important to remember that kids' curiosity is generative, supercharging their brain development as they seek to understand this amazing world they've landed in.

At some point, most of us stop asking so many questions. And the questions we do ask become more procedural than *wonder*-ful: *Where did I put my purse? When is my doctor's appointment? Who is on pick-up this afternoon? What did the dog just eat? Can I put the kids to bed yet?* But even when we feel trapped by the needs of the day, compelling questions are still out there waiting for us.

You'll remember that Keltner and his team found that "big ideas" were a common source of awe for adults—and that the definition of awe includes encountering something vast. That vastness is not limited to landscapes. We also encounter vast *concepts*.

Cognitive Accommodation

Awe is more than an emotion of the heart; it also improves our thinking. That's because *cognitive accommodation* is a feature of awe. This term stems from Jean Piaget's theory of cognitive development.

Put simply, when we learn something new, we alter or expand our existing mental schemas to make room for it.

Young kids practice cognitive accommodation all the time. Think of a toddler whose only experience with dogs is the family's small Shih Tzu. One day, the child meets the neighbor's Great Dane. Wow! The child's mental concept of "dog" quickly expands to include more shapes and sizes.

Cognitive accommodation is at the heart of good education: It is what allows students to build on prior knowledge to revise, expand, and deepen their understanding of a concept. As Summer Allen wrote in the "Science of Awe" white paper: "Awe's ability to elicit cognitive accommodation may also explain why humans evolved to experience this unique emotion. Experiencing awe may be adaptive because it encourages us to take in new information and adjust our mental structures around this information, helping us navigate our world."[2]

The Awe-Curiosity Connection

It is no surprise, then, that awe is linked to children's academic performance.[3] If I had to turn the research into an oversimplified visual, it would look like this:

Awe → Curiosity → Learning → Memory

This all leads to greater academic outcomes.

"One of my favorite findings suggests that awe might help spur curiosity about the world," psychologist Craig Anderson told me. Anderson was part of a team that studied how this emotion influenced teenagers. "The more awe they felt, the more curiosity they expressed and the better they performed in school," he said.

Awe is sometimes described as a "knowledge emotion." Paul Silvia, a psychology professor at the University of North Carolina, Greensboro, describes knowledge emotions as "a family of emotional states that foster learning, exploring, and reflecting." These emotions include surprise, interest, confusion, and awe and stem from experiences that are "unexpected, complicated, and mentally challenging, and they motivate learning in its broadest sense."[4]

According to Silvia, awe is a powerful educational tool because it motivates people to explore things that stretch their understanding of the world. He wrote, "When people see beautiful and striking color images of supernovas, black holes, and planetary nebulas, they usually report feelings of awe and wonder. These feelings then motivate them to learn about what they are seeing and their scientific importance."[5]

When You Wonder, You're Learning

None of this research would surprise Fred Rogers, for whom wonder was pedagogy. He knew that curiosity is what primes children's brains for learning. He also had this incredible capacity to communicate his own wonder through the screen.

I reached out to Gregg Behr and Ryan Rydzewski, coauthors of *When You Wonder, You're Learning: Mister Rogers' Enduring Lessons for Raising Creative, Curious, Caring Kids*, to hear more about what they learned from studying Rogers's work. Here is what they told me:

> When Fred Rogers sang the words "When you wonder, you're learning," he wasn't kidding. In a very real sense, he was right. We know from modern science that when we're in a state of wonder, something switches on in the brain. We start to absorb all kinds of information. And the more curiosity we feel, the more likely we are to retain that information.
>
> Think about it this way: If someone hands you a textbook on dendrology (the scientific study of trees), you probably won't rush home to read it. But what if, instead, that person gives you *The Hidden Life of Trees* by Peter Wohlleben, promising that you'll learn all sorts of secrets about how trees talk to one another? You're much more likely to learn from the book that makes you

curious. That's why some scientists think that curiosity may be just as important as intelligence when it comes to children's success in school.

According to researchers, curiosity has a "fundamental impact on learning and memory."[6] When kids are curious, they are more motivated to learn and more adept at retaining information. Think about a four-year-old who knows the name of every dinosaur, a ten-year-old who can recite and explain the g-forces of dozens of roller coasters, or a fourteen-year-old who has memorized every *Hamilton* lyric. No teacher has assigned this work. The four-year-old went to a natural history museum and was mesmerized by the enormous skeletons. The ten-year-old rode their first roller coaster and became fascinated by the feeling and the physics of it all. The fourteen-year-old had never heard a musical, or history, quite like this one, so they kept on listening. Awe, curiosity, learning, memory.

Here is another fantastic finding: Curiosity has an amplifying effect on *other* learning. One study out of the University of California, Davis, found that when participants were curious about the initial information presented to them, they could then more easily absorb unrelated information.[7] Simply being in a curious state of mind helped participants' brains memorize material that they were less excited about. As the study's lead author, Matthias Gruber, said, "Curiosity may put the brain in a state that allows it to learn and retain any kind of information, like a vortex that sucks in what you are motivated to learn, and also everything around it."[8]

This is news parents can use. Engaging with kids' big questions and helping them discover what sparks their curiosity is a concrete way to support their learning in general. The challenge is not to make them fall in love with *all* subjects. But what if we nurtured their curiosity with one or two? What if we paid close attention to what sparked their interest, what inspired their awe, and nudged it along?

I remember a fourth grader I taught in New Jersey years ago. He was obsessed with roller coasters and had amassed an encyclopedic knowledge of rides around the world. His eyes sparkled when he explained negative g-force—or airtime—to me. But he was *not* as thrilled about writing lessons. His dashed-off paragraphs were a stark contrast to his loquacious conversation. So I invited him to write a book about roller coasters, to teach me and his classmates what he knew. His eyes lit up. A month later, he had composed a lengthy booklet detailing his favorite rides.

This story does not end with him becoming a structural engineer. Evan Goldstein recently completed a Ph.D. in modern Jewish literature and is now a religious studies professor.

I sent Evan an out-of-the-blue email with a couple questions: Did he have any memory of this fourth-grade fascination? What had captured his curiosity since that time? His thorough response brought tears to my eyes. Teachers interact with kids for such a small slice of their lives. We hope we have been a pebble in their pond and our influence continues to ripple. But our memories of them are often frozen in time. Reading Evan's response was an experience with cognitive accommodation— expanding my perception of a beloved former student.

He described how, as a kid, he tended to get fascinated with particular things, including roller coasters. He pored through almanacs and world records books and committed thousands of facts to memory just for the joy of it. In high school, his curiosity led him to study the Supreme Court—not just the rulings but "the oral arguments, with all their ritual and strange code and cadence of speech." This led him to initially study politics in college, which eventually pointed him toward studying religion and its "questions of cosmic significance." As he concluded:

> That's probably too neat a line to draw between roller coasters and Jewish modernism. But I really do believe that something

like awe is the whole point of education. I did a quick search, and it seems like "awe" is a viable, maybe even better, translation for the Hebrew word *yirat*—which is usually translated as "fear." So Proverbs 1:7 could be read as: "The *awe* of the Lord is the beginning of wisdom."

Asking Better Questions

Awe is also linked to another C-word that supports our children's academic growth: *creativity*. Multiple studies have found a direct link between awe and creative thinking.[9] And it makes sense, since awe prompts us to reexamine and reevaluate. Similarly, creativity requires us to ask questions, see possibilities, and think about things in new ways. As philosophy professor Helen De Cruz writes, "Awe increases our tolerance for uncertainty and opens our receptivity to new and unusual ideas."[10] A study from Keltner's lab found that "simply watching short videos of expansive images of the Earth leads people to come up with more original examples when asked to name items from a certain category (e.g., 'furniture')."[11]

One form of creativity is simply asking good questions. Warren Berger is a self-described "questionologist" and author of the book *A More Beautiful Question*. In his work as a journalist, Berger noticed something in common about the creative innovators he interviewed. They asked really good questions. He writes, "We're all hungry today for better answers. But first, we must learn to ask the right questions."[12] On this front, our children can often be our teachers.

In a blog post on his website, Berger tells the story of three-year-old Jennifer and her inventor father, Edwin Land.[13] In 1943, Land was taking photographs and his young daughter wanted to know why she couldn't see the pictures immediately. "Why do we have to wait?" she asked. It would have been easy for Land to dismiss the question as childish; everyone knew that it took time to get film developed. But instead, he embraced her query as a puzzle she had set for him. Five years later, Land invented the Polaroid Instant camera.

What I love most about this story is this: Land took his kid's question seriously. Amazing things happen when we grapple with big, seemingly unsolvable problems—and when we allow kids to grapple with them too.

Take this awe-inducing story: In 2023, Michelle Blouin Williams, a math teacher at St. Mary's Academy in New Orleans, asked her high schoolers a question with an impossible answer. As a bonus on a math contest, she challenged students to create a new proof for the Pythagorean theorem using trigonometry. She didn't expect success— what she was looking for was simply "some ingenuity."

Two of her students, seniors Calcea Johnson and Ne'Kiya Jackson, embraced the challenge. For two months, they used most of their free time—and reams of paper—working on this problem. And then they solved it. According to the *60 Minutes* segment on the young women's feat, "There had been more than three hundred documented proofs of the Pythagorean Theorem using algebra and geometry, but for two thousand years a proof using trigonometry was thought to be impossible." After they presented their proof at a conference, the news "blew up," according to Jackson. They even got a shout-out from Michelle Obama and a key to the city.

When asked why she thought the story went viral, Jackson responded, "Probably because we're African American, one. And we're also women. . . . Oh, and our age." But, she added, "I'd like to actually be celebrated for what it is. It's a great mathematical achievement."[14]

Whenever I hear a story like this, I wonder if we routinely underestimate our kids. Heather Hill, an education professor at Harvard University, told me that "there's heaps of evidence that kids are naturally very creative when it comes to mathematics." In the same way that kids create their own stories or make up songs, "kids will invent their own methods for solving mathematics problems, even problems that are sometimes very complex." As she told me, simply "asking mathematical questions is a form of creativity."

You probably haven't developed a new mathematical proof, but have you ever spent days, months, or even years inspired by a question? Have you ever seen your child get blissfully lost in exploring a big idea? Last year, my daughter spent months researching the diamond industry: Why does one little rock create so much human and environmental devastation? Who decided that this rock was the most valuable one, anyway? What could we do now to right these wrongs? My son is currently enamored by this question: Is the Tasmanian tiger really extinct? Could a small number still be out there, somewhere?

In a podcast with the John Templeton Foundation, Keltner noted that wonder is a mental state where you seek to figure out what just gave you that feeling of awe. "You're testing hypotheses and formulating questions and gathering data and just making sense of what was vast and mysterious that gave you this feeling of awe," he said. "Rainbows blew the minds of Newton and Descartes. How in the world could light come through a water molecule and produce the color spectrum? And those guys—from that feeling of awe at the mysteries of rainbows— entered into an enduring state of wonder."[15] And from there, they used their scientific skills to find the answers.

One of my favorite examples of awe leading to curiosity leading to learning comes from Robin Wall Kimmerer, a Potawatomi botanist and author of *Braiding Sweetgrass: Indigenous Wisdom, Scientific Knowledge, and the Teachings of Plants.* Here was her question: Why do aster and goldenrod look so beautiful together?

It's a lovely question—one I could imagine my daughter asking me as a flower-loving preschooler. But is it scientific? For Kimmerer, yes. After all, these vibrant yellow and purple flowers grow in clusters in the autumn. Where you find one, you often find the other. For her professors, though, Kimmerer's question was not so scientific.

Kimmerer describes how there was little room for questions of aesthetics and emotions in her science classes. And yet there *is* a scientific purpose to these flowers keeping company: Purple and yellow are complementary colors—not just for human eyes but also for bee eyes. So when asters and goldenrods keep each other company, they attract more pollinators than they would by themselves. As Kimmerer writes: "The question of goldenrod and aster was of course just emblematic of what I really wanted to know. It was an architecture of relationships, of connections that I yearned to understand. I wanted to see the shimmering threads that hold it all together. And I wanted to know why we love the world, why the most ordinary scrap of meadow can rock us back on our heels in awe."[16]

One of the simplest ways parents can encourage kids to ask great questions is to ask better questions ourselves. Educators at Harvard University's Project Zero offer several suggestions for posing questions to kids that invite both curiosity and creativity.[17] I've modified these for parents:

- Ask kids questions that invite imaginative and divergent thinking: "What might happen if . . .?"

- Ask open-ended questions that normalize uncertainty and let kids explore possibilities. It's the difference between asking, "What are the phases of the moon?" and "What have you noticed about the moon?"

- Observe your children's interests, play, and conversations to figure out what they are wondering about. Use those to develop questions that take their learning deeper.

- Invite kids to share their wonder. Take their questions seriously. Make a Wonder Wall listing things your family wants to learn more about.

Transcendent Thinking

Remember the kindergartner who wondered, *How do people grow?* That child so perfectly captured a central mystery of parenthood: How do we help our children grow? Every age is a stage, and every stage is an opportunity to witness and encourage growth.

Take mid-adolescence, approximately ages fourteen to eighteen, for example. At this stage of life, the teen brain develops an increased capacity for "transcendent thinking." Teens can move beyond the here-and-now to think about complex systems, ethical implications, and social dynamics in more profound ways. As researchers from University of Southern California (USC) put it, teens develop the capacity to "invoke broader perspectives on themselves, other people, and social systems, and draw on cultural values and associated emotions to infer social and ethical implications and build deeper understandings."[18]

These USC researchers launched a five-year study. They asked a group of fourteen- to eighteen-year-olds of color living in low-income urban communities to listen to and reflect on real-life stories from teens around the world. All the teens in the study exhibited some degree of transcendent thinking, but some teens showed a greater capacity than others. And that, in turn, had long-term benefits. As the study found, when teens spent more time grappling with the ethical implications of the stories, this transcendent thinking "predicted future increases in the coordination of two key brain networks: the default-mode network, involved in reflective, autobiographical, and free-form thinking, and the executive control network, involved in effortful, focused thinking," regardless of participants' IQs or socioeconomic statuses. The study continues, "This neural development predicted late-adolescent identity development, which predicted young-adult self-liking and relationship satisfaction."

Put more simply, your child *will* develop transcendent-thinking skills as a teenager; leaning into these skills may enhance their brain coordination in ways that benefit their self-concept and their relationships with others. That's a strong argument for engaging teens with compelling ideas, meaningful questions, and real conversation. I think teens of every generation get a lot of unfair grief about being shallow or self-centered, but that just hasn't been my experience (and it likely hasn't been yours)—especially when you talk to them one-on-one. If four-year-olds are wired to understand their new world, fourteen-year-olds are wired to find their place in it.

MJ's and Kate's Stories

What does a teen's transcendent thinking sound like? Let me introduce you to two high school seniors, MJ "Vinny" Worsley and Kate Novack, whose minds travel to wondrous places, and who share their stories in their own words.

MJ

In the dawn of my junior year, all I could think about was the Arctic and the Franklin Expedition. Even in the boiling Texas sun—running with my gangly-legged dog straining at her leash, both of us grinning and gasping in the oven-hot August air—that polar expedition was under my skin, flowing through my head. This isn't the first time that some or another subject has taken over my brain—the list includes Patient H. M., etymology, photography, Amazonian snakes, Minkowski, and medieval Nordic runes. I lost a week of sleep because I couldn't stop thinking about American Sign Language.

How can I explain how happy this makes me, or why? How can I explain to my friends why I wrote seven painstaking pages of meteorological information just to have one beloved paragraph detailing the Franklin Expedition?

It's the human part of it that gets me every time. The fact that humanity, past and present, is always wandering to the edge of the map, all that beauty in the horror. Even aboard the doomed Franklin

Expedition, people wrote poetry. The sailors, the captains, the lost and the buried—they all had bad dreams and good ones, hangnails, sweethearts, sunsets, and doubts. They sang, shivered, and sweat while history churned around them.

Isn't that beautiful? It's what I search for in all my amateur research. That ache. That inexorable pull in the knowledge that we explore and learn and love and die, and it's all melted together, it's all so beautiful. The men of the Franklin Expedition were doomed, just like you and I, to be tragically human. I don't know how not to fall in love with that.

Kate

In every class, I was the student asking the *why*—behind a character's motivation in a novel, the solution to a complex mathematical problem, or the decision of a historical figure.

On the first day of my junior year philosophy class, my teacher began with, "You are not a good student of philosophy if you are not constantly asking questions and seeking to learn their answers." I felt so gratified in that moment knowing that I found an outlet for learning where I could be comfortable in the uncomfortable.

I like Aristotle, which might be surprising for a seventeen-year-old high school senior. I am fascinated with a philosopher who lived almost two thousand years ago because of my desire to answer the kind of big questions he asks. I wonder, *What is my purpose, my telos?*

While such questions can intimidate, I find that they enhance my curiosity and excitement for learning and discovery. Pondering philosophical ideas helps me discern what to do when I don't know what to do. It's not about always having all the answers; it's about the questions and the search for meaning, beauty, and truth.

Breaking Down the Myths and Silos

When my son told me the other day that he "didn't really like math," I laughed to myself. He had just spent most of the day poring over NBA shooting percentages, examining player stats on his baseball cards, and building a marble run—all math activities.

My scientist dad adored the 1959 Disney cartoon *Donald in Mathmagic Land*. Math is everywhere, he'd tell me. It's in the shape of a spider's web, the size of a shadow, and the swirl of a seashell. He knew that science and math aren't just subjects in school, they are a way of understanding the world.

Math is everywhere—and so are art, literature, science. But adults and kids tend to silo subjects. Think of how a middle or high schooler's day is typically arranged: They travel from math to English to social studies to science, as if these are disparate and unrelated fields. It becomes easy to view the arts/humanities and STEM (science, technology, engineering, and mathematics) as separate ways of knowing. Our culture also propagates overly simplistic theories about right versus left brain and "learning styles" that unwittingly give kids a sense that their brains simply aren't wired to learn some things.

However, as we covered in chapter 3, both artists and engineers need spatial reasoning skills and the ability to recognize patterns. Mathematicians, photographers, and painters use geometry in their work—including shapes, symmetry, and measurement. Music is built on physics, ratio, and proportion.

Sometimes, kids see themselves as either an "arts person" or a "math person"—as if they can't be both. And I can't tell you the number of times I've heard parents overtly, though well-meaningly, confirm this type of fixed thinking, often reflecting their own struggles of not being "good at math" (or art or whatever subject).

While it can feel as if our skills are set in stone, we know that is simply not true. I also know how hard it can be to explain this to a kid who's struggling in a particular school subject. One of my favorite books for middle schoolers is Barbara Oakley and Terrence Sejnowski's *Learning How to Learn: How to Succeed in School Without Spending All Your Time Studying*. Oakley's professional biography does not suggest that she was once a struggling math and science student. After all, she is an engineering professor. But Oakley described herself to me as a "former math flunky" who "retooled" her brain after years of thinking she just wasn't good at STEM subjects. She has since made it her life's work to help others "learn how to learn" by explaining some key principles from neuroscience to kids. Oakley said that when we teach children and teens *how* they learn, we can blow open their sense of possibility. "I tell students, you don't just have to be stuck following your passion. You can *broaden* your passions enormously. And that can have enormous implications for how your life unfolds. We always say *follow your passions*, but sometimes that locks people into focusing on what comes easily or what they are already good at. You can get passionate about—and good at—many things!"

That is true for parents too. What if we modeled learning and doing things outside of our *I'm good at this* comfort zone? What if we were walking examples of *I didn't think I could, but then I did*? It may seem like a small thing, but I started boxing classes a couple of months ago. I have been guilty of telling my kids that I'm not particularly "sporty." My participation in team sports ended with fourth grade softball. But a friend dragged me to a boxing class with her, and I was hooked. Was I coordinated the first week? Nope. I'm still mastering jab, cross, hook combos. And I love telling my kids about it—about what I'm learning and how good it feels. Boxing has expanded my concept of what my body can do.

The Upside of Struggle

Learning isn't all sunshine and roses for any of us. Kids often struggle to feel awe when they are frustrated with a task and doubt their own ability to learn a subject. And yet, paradoxically, we are often profoundly inspired when we hear about how *other* people struggled on their journeys to success.

A few years ago, I came across some fascinating research about teens and science.[19] Columbia University researchers posed this question to ninth and tenth graders in New York City: What kind of people can become scientists? Almost every student gave empowering responses, such as "People who work hard" or "Anyone who seems interested in the field of science." But despite these beliefs, many of these same teens struggled to imagine *themselves* as scientists, citing concerns such as "I'm not good at science" and "Even if I work hard, I will not do well." So what could help change this mindset?

The study found that teens who read about scientists' personal and intellectual struggles were more motivated to learn science. That's because students often view scientific ability as a fixed trait—something you are born with that can't be changed. Either you have it or you don't. But when students learned how even accomplished scientists struggled, they began to see that challenges are simply part of what it means to be a scientist. Now, that's a *big idea*—one powerful enough to change their perception of themselves as students. The effect was especially pronounced for lower-performing students for whom "exposure to struggle stories led to significantly better science-class performance than low-performing students who read achievement stories."

I love this research, particularly for our kids who struggle with aspects of academic learning. Jeffrey Mitchell is the Head of School at Currey Ingram Academy, a school in Tennessee for students with learning differences. He told me that creating awe is the "Mount Olympus of educational outcomes." Because awe is such a powerful learning tool, he said, "it is fair and useful to ask how to get students who have been demoralized in the educational process to feel awe."

Mitchell says he is guided by three principles:

1. Truly *embrace*—not just accept—every child for who they are as an individual human being.

2. Use research-based teaching methods to build *foundational* cognitive skills. When kids have these skills, it helps them pursue the questions that excite their imagination.

3. Find ways to systematically identify and showcase the strengths of every child.

I find each of Mitchell's principles equally applicable to parenting: Look for ways to celebrate your kid's strengths, particularly if they are struggling with aspects of school. Pay attention to their interests and skills—from technology to skateboarding to anime—and explore ways they can use these interests to strengthen other areas of their life.

This stuff isn't fluff. Curiosity can help kids navigate academic difficulties. In a study of dyslexic Nobel Laureates and prominent scholars, researchers found that these thinkers "were able to persist in their efforts to read because they were motivated to explore an early and ardent interest."[20] Another study found that interest in a topic is a more powerful predictor of future success in a field than grades.[21]

Awe and Intellectual Humility

During a recent piano lesson, my kid began to rush through a piece, ignoring the new, more difficult fingering. The teacher paused the lesson and said, "Do you know what it takes to be a great pianist? Humility. You have to acknowledge when something is hard. That is a strength. You must be humble enough to say, *I'm not good at this yet. I need help. It's going to take a lot of effort and practice.* That is how you grow."

Just as awe is underrated as an emotion, intellectual humility is undervalued as a character trait. We know from the research that one outcome of awe is a feeling of humility because it helps you remember your small place in a large and wondrous universe. So how is humility helpful for kids?

I reached out to Tenelle Porter. Porter has spent her academic career studying intellectual humility, which she defines as "recognizing the limits of your knowledge and valuing the insight of someone else." Being humble does not mean a child is insecure. In fact, according to Porter's research, "intellectually humble students were more motivated to learn and more likely to use effective metacognitive strategies, like quizzing themselves to check their own understanding."[22] Kids who recognized the limitations of their knowledge were also more likely to "persist with a difficult task, accept feedback, and learn from disagreement" than their less humble peers.

As Porter told me, "You can't learn what you think you already know. Without intellectual humility, we're stuck where we are—we're stuck with our current knowledge, current mistakes, current misunderstandings. Only when we're willing to acknowledge that we don't have everything figured out can we really learn and grow." Awe often reminds us about how much we don't yet fully understand. Instead of getting defensive about what we don't know, humility opens us up to learning more.

One of the best ways to nurture kids' intellectual humility is to model it yourself. "Admit it when you don't know something, own it when you're mistaken, reveal it if you're confused," said Porter. This can be hard to do. You may worry that your kids will lose confidence in you if you don't have all the answers. But Porter's research found that adult humility is a powerful tool. When we model intellectual humility, our kids "become more comfortable doing it too."

I like to imagine a future where people were more attuned to life's mysteries and beauty—and more willing to admit their limitations and learn from others. As Kimmerer wrote, "Doing science with awe and humility is a powerful act of reciprocity with the more-than-human world."[23]

Making Room for Hobbies

Have you ever noticed that your kids can be incredibly busy yet also seem to be just going through the motions in their activities and schoolwork? Overprogramming does not necessarily beget curiosity, creativity, and wonder, and it leaves little room for asking and exploring big questions.

Every time I talk to a high-achieving, stressed-out teen or read another story about the pediatric mental health crisis, I think of these words from my interview with Dacher Keltner. They read like a poem, so I'm taking the liberty to structure them as such.

> How do you find awe?
> You allow unstructured time.
> How do you find awe?
> You wander. You drift through.
> You take a walk with no aim.
> How do you find awe?
> You slow things down.
> You allow for mystery and open questions
> rather than test-driven answers.
> You allow people to engage
> in the humanities
> of dance and visual art and music.

When we allow our kids to "wander"—to follow their questions, to dabble in this and that—we create space for them to stumble upon awe. I love watching kids drift toward and away from hobbies, evolving as they discover what speaks to them. Think of a teen who moves from consuming fantasy books to writing fanfiction to running a D&D club. Reading sparks an interest; fanfiction taps into this teen's latent creativity and connects them to a wider community; D&D forges friendships with creative peers who want to build worlds together.

Keltner's wisdom also reminds me of Michele Borba's research. Borba is a child development expert and author of *Thrivers: The Surprising Reasons Why Some Kids Struggle and Others Shine*. She spent months interviewing thousands of teens, and one of the clear messages that came through was this: "Thrivers have hobbies—they have something they can decompress to."[24] But here's the catch. When she asked teens, "What are your hobbies?" they often replied, "What's a hobby? We don't have enough time for hobbies." Their lives, she told me, had become full of "should dos" instead of "want to dos."

Purposeful activities are restorative for kids. Have you ever gotten so into an activity you love that time that time seemed to fly by? That's called being in a state of "flow." Mihaly Csikszentmihalyi, the psychologist who coined the term, defined it as "a state in which people are so involved in an activity that nothing else seems to matter."[25] You feel a joy and energizing focus that transforms your sense of time. We sometimes also talk about this as being "in the zone." Csikszentmihalyi believed that our most cherished memories don't come from passive or relaxing times, though those can be both delightful and necessary. Rather, he wrote, "The best moments usually occur if a person's body or mind is stretched to its limits in a voluntary effort to accomplish something difficult and worthwhile."[26]

So how do we help our kids find purposeful, worthwhile activities that help them experience that flow? I think it's helpful to remember this: Kids' interests will evolve—sometimes rapidly—and that's usually a good thing! And their interests may not align with ours or with our sense of what they *should* be doing—nor do they need to.

When my kids were young, I was the driving force behind most of their extracurricular activities, signing them up for Girl Scouts here and a tumbling class there. That began to shift during the tweenage years. For example, last year my daughter dropped piano lessons. Never mind that I had repeatedly told both my kids that piano lessons until eighth grade was nonnegotiable. It turns out it was negotiable, particularly when an astute piano teacher turned and said, "You are such a good and diligent piano student, but it's clear your heart isn't in it. Is this how you want to spend your time?" The answer was a resounding "No!"

So what occupies her free time now? Creative writing, acting in a community drama troupe, track practice, and filling up lots and lots of sketchbooks. This summer, she has also taken to waking up at dawn to take morning walks, often photographing the wildlife that also rises with the sun. My husband and I recently marveled that 100 percent of these activities are driven by her.

While it's a great feeling as a parent to see your kid pursue an activity that is meaningful for them, it's also a dance, because often kids won't discover an interest unless someone introduces it to them and encourages them through the initial struggle of learning something new. My son asked to quit piano when his sibling did, but I told him to give it one more year. He said to me the other day, "I'm so glad you didn't let me quit piano when [my sister] did. I love it so much now! Can I learn how to DJ too?"

So do we let our kids quit soccer after a frustrating practice or hang up their tap shoes if they're struggling to get a combo right? Isn't it our job to keep them engaged in these activities? Why did I let one child quit piano and encourage the other one to continue? Borba told me that a good guiding question for parents is this: Who is doing the pushing and pulling?

She pointed me toward the work of psychologist Benjamin Bloom. Bloom studied the lives of accomplished mathematicians, athletes, and musicians, and he found that adults usually introduced them to these activities when they were young. But—and it's a big *but*—before long, the child was pulling the parent.[27] As adults, we should "periodically step back and ask, *Who is doing the pulling?*" Borba said. "And if you are the one always pulling [your kid] to put on their soccer cleats or practice the piano, maybe they are telling you something." Maybe it's no longer a source of wonder and satisfaction. Thankfully, our kids' worlds are brimming with possibilities.

One way to spark kids' wonder is to introduce various new activities—without expectations. Just *exploration*. For example:

- a one-off online or rec center class
- a morning of birdwatching
- a knitting lesson with a grandparent over Zoom
- a trial martial arts class
- an origami or manga YouTube tutorial
- a morning volunteering at a farm
- an outing with a teenage neighbor who knows how to geocache
- a local theater performance

"When [your kids] find something beyond your scope, find them a mentor," said Borba. "It doesn't have to be pricey—it might be the neighbor next door. We are not partnering with other parents nearly enough."

Borba also suggests parents become curious observers of their kids' curiosity, asking questions like *What activities ignite my kid's imagination? What gives them an extra spark of joy? What increases their confidence, reduces their stress, or helps them enjoy their own company?* "Find out what helps your child be the best version of themselves," said Borba. And then give them the freedom to pursue those activities.

My dad excelled at both piquing my curiosity and changing course as my interests changed. He was the one who got me a college geology textbook when I was a nine-year-old who loved rocks. The one who brought home Petri dishes so we could "grow things." The one who woke me up in the middle of the night to watch that meteor shower. The one who took me out to lunch at the only sushi restaurant in town when I expressed interest in Japan. The one who read every article I wrote for the school newspaper. The one who searched for used child psychology textbooks at the bookstore when I announced that I wanted to be a teacher. The one who wrote (but never published) a children's book about the wonder of gravity. I love that my son— named for the grandpa he never met—got a Most Inquisitive award at his end-of-school class ceremony this year.

A Final Thought

On the last day of fourth grade, my son brought home a report he had written on physicist Stephen Hawking. This child (the same one who called me to his room to ask about the edge of the universe at age six) had spent weeks studying Hawking and his research. I got goosebumps when I read his conclusion:

> There are some questions that everybody wonders. Some of them are related to you, like *How do I do this?*, and other ones relate to the world, like *Where did we come from?*
>
> People like Darwin have answered the big questions of how humans and animals evolved, but one person tried to answer where *everything* came from. That man was Stephen Hawking. Hawking is known worldwide as a person that represents success through adversity. He was diagnosed with ALS at age twenty-one, and he later stated that being told that he was going to die really made him realize that life is worth living, and that he was going to live it.
>
> Stephen Hawking's discoveries and theories have impacted how scientists look at the universe on one level. On a personal level, he inspires me to never give up, no matter what challenges or questions I might encounter. Against all odds, Hawking has left his mark on the world. Hawking famously stated: "I want to inspire the next generation to look up at the stars, and not down at their feet."

I agree with Hawking, while also recognizing that it's often my kids who help me look up from my feet (or my phone) to stare at something grander. When they were young, their questions about the world helped me experience it anew. As they get older, their questions challenge my assumptions. I have the awesome privilege of accompanying them as they make discoveries about themselves, the world, and their place in it.

5 Wonderful Ways to Explore Big Ideas with Kids

1. Read About It. Go to the library and challenge your kids to find books that spark their curiosity for any reason: books about volcanos, mythology, sports statistics, inventors, dinosaurs, the ocean, puppies, baking, or the cosmos. Go to a bookstore and just explore. Sometimes, flipping through the pages is enough to inspire more questions and more understanding of the world.

2. Let's Find Out. When children pose a question we can't answer, here's a powerful response: "That's a great question! Let's find out." Experiment together. Look it up in a book or online. Call a friend or family member who is an expert. All these activities show them their questions are valued and that there are tools for finding answers.

3. Listen Up. One way to support kids' and teens' wonder is simply this: Listen to their questions. It feels good when people pay attention to us. When we honor kids' questions, it validates their curiosity and invites them to keep exploring. Fred Rogers wrote, "It's what *you* bring to the children every day—your listening, your caring, your enthusiasm, and your responding to their ideas, thoughts, and feelings—that encourages and inspires children to ask questions and be imaginative."[28]

4. Question Mirroring. When you're at the beach and your kid asks, "Why does the ocean change colors?" instead of answering immediately or jumping on your phone, send the question back to them. "Why do *you* think it does?" As parents, we often feel a need to have all the answers—but when we unlock our children's wonder, they are apt to ask questions we've never thought of.

5. What If . . . ? One of my favorite questions that kids ask is often an unspoken one: *What will happen if . . . ?* This is a great scientific question that helps kids understand cause and effect. Of course, these questions can also be messy as kids wonder, *What will happen if I drop this egg on the floor?* or *What will happen if I flush my toothbrush down the toilet?* When necessary, try redirecting their experiments without squelching their curiosity. If they want to know what drawing on walls is like, get some bathtub paint and set them loose in the tub. In other words, try saying, "You can't do that, but you can do this!"

10 Picture Books to Inspire Big Ideas

Happy Dreamer **by Peter H. Reynolds.** There are so many ways to dream big. This book follows a young protagonist who embraces their unique way of seeing the world and finds joy in imaginative pursuits.

You Wonder All the Time **by Deborah Farmer Kris and Jennifer Zivoin.** "Where do colors go at night, and why do shadows creep?" Drawn from real questions from the author's kids, *You Wonder All the Time* affirms children's innate curiosity.

National Geographic Kids Almanac. Every year, *National Geographic* publishes an almanac for kids that is brimming with facts on just about every subject: geography, animals, sports, weather, astronomy, and many more. A great resource for all the fact-loving kids in your life.

The Girl with Big, Big Questions **by Britney Winn Lee and Jacob Souva.** "Why can't people live on the moon?" "Can I be president when I grow up?" "What makes a person good?" This girl has big questions and is relentless in pursuing answers.

Digging for Words: José Alberto Gutiérrez and the Library He Built **by Angela Burke Kunkel and Paola Escobar.** This book tells the true story of José Alberto Gutiérrez's journey from garbage collector to library founder in Colombia. Collecting discarded books, he established a library, offering hope and education to his community.

Loujain Dreams of Sunflowers **by Uma Mishra-Newbery, Lina Al-Hathloul, and Rebecca Green.** Loujain is a young girl who longs to fly, but in her land, only boys are allowed to attach their wings. But she is determined to see the sunflowers her Baba has told her about. The story is inspired by the real-life Loujain Al-Hathloul, who was imprisoned in Saudi Arabia for driving and successfully led the fight to lift the ban on women drivers.

Twenty Questions **by Mac Barnett and Christian Robinson.** The author poses twenty questions—some profound, all playful, and none of which have definitive answers. Answering even one of these questions can take kids on an imaginative journey.

A Stone Is a Story **by Leslie Barnard Booth and Marc Martin.** Booth tells the geologic story of planet Earth, using a small stone that you can hold in your hand. A great reminder that even the most ordinary objects have incredible stories.

The Girl Who Thought in Pictures: The Story of Dr. Temple Grandin **by Julia Finley Mosca and Daniel Rieley.** This book depicts the life of Dr. Temple Grandin, an autistic woman who revolutionized the understanding of animal behavior. Grandin embraced her unique thinking style to become a renowned scientist and an advocate for autism awareness.

Noticing **by Kobi Yamada and Elise Hurst.** The note from the author captures the heart of his book: "My hope is that *Noticing* will spark readers' imaginations to dream, believe, and wonder about all the extraordinary possibilities that are waiting to be discovered . . . I believe the more we look for the good, the more we find it, and that approach can lead to a richer understanding of the world, ourselves, and each other."

CHAPTER FIVE

THE WONDER OF BELONGING

What should young people do with their lives today? Many things, obviously. But the most daring thing is to create stable communities in which the terrible disease of loneliness can be cured.

—Kurt Vonnegut

Loneliness is headline news. In May 2023, US Surgeon General Vivek Murthy declared loneliness a public health epidemic.[1] Also in 2023, a Meta-Gallup survey of more than 140 countries found that almost 25 percent of the world's population felt "fairly or very lonely."[2] And according to a 2024 American Psychiatric Association (APA) poll, the group most likely to experience this emotion were young adults (people ages eighteen to thirty-four), 30 percent of whom said they were "lonely every day or several times a week."[3] Today's kids are growing up into lonely young adults. And let's face it: Parenting can be a lonely business too.

The APA poll used this definition of *loneliness*: "feeling like you do not have meaningful or close relationships or a sense of belonging."

Close, meaningful relationships. Belonging. We need this connection across the lifespan, obviously. But think back to, say, your middle school days—how much you craved belonging, how intoxicating it was to make a new friend who really got you, how alive you felt when you found your place on a team, club, or performance group.

Awe researchers have found that "collective effervescence" is one of the top sources of awe.[4] It's a fancy term for a rich emotional experience. Coined by Émile Durkheim in 1912, *collective effervescence* describes the feeling of working together in harmony toward a common goal. Think of an a cappella group singing together, creating spine-tingling resonance. Think of a basketball team where the players seem to sense where their teammates will be on the court before they get there. Think of a sweaty group of teens who spent the day helping build a house for Habitat for Humanity.

Kids crave being part of a group. They are also in a developmental state of self-focus, particularly in early adolescence. Moments of collective effervescence, of belonging, help them feel less insular and more connected to others. Psychologist Fan Yang describes awe as a "self-transcendent" emotion. That's precisely what makes it so special, she told me. "Compared to other positive emotions such as happiness and pride, awe has a unique power to make us feel smaller and see our position in the bigger context of the world and life."

Collective Neuroscience, or "I was just thinking the same thing!"

On a recent family group chat, I responded to a comment with a picture of a dancing chicken. "AH! I WAS JUST ABOUT TO SEND THAT EXACT SAME GIF," one kid replied. Moments like this happen a lot in our family and probably in yours too. We find ourselves singing the same song, having the same reactions, and finishing each other's sentences. A new field of research has been studying this phenomenon: collective neuroscience. Durkheim may have coined the term *collective effervescence* over a hundred years ago, but modern neuroscience is offering a new dimension to it.

Here's the simple rundown: Traditionally, brain research has focused on one brain at a time. But humans are social creatures. We like to be with other people, and when we work together, we often come up with better ideas than we do on our own. Scientists have discovered that when people talk or share an experience, their brain waves synchronize. According to an article in *Scientific American*: "In classrooms where students are engaged with the teacher, for example, their patterns of brain processing begin to align with that teacher's—and greater alignment may mean better learning. Neural waves in certain brain regions of people listening to a musical performance match those of the performer—the greater the synchrony, the greater the enjoyment. Couples exhibit higher degrees of brain synchrony than nonromantic pairs, as do close friends compared with more distant acquaintances."[5]

The article also shares that "neurons in corresponding locations of the different brains fire at the same time, creating matching patterns, like dancers moving together." I love that image. So does Marinda, a sixteen-year-old from Wisconsin who told me that "dancers moving together" is, quite literally, her most potent source of awe. "Every year, I dance in my studio's annual *Nutcracker* ballet. We practice for months to get the choreography just right, and we rely on years' worth of training to execute the moves and storyline precisely," she said. "When I'm not dancing, I like to watch. It's this awesome feeling of seeing something we've all worked so hard for finally come together. And I get to experience this every year!"

Kids Want to Belong

Belonging doesn't just happen. Take Marinda's story, for example. Her parents support her desire to dance. Together, they found a studio that nurtures its dancers. Marinda found a group of peers who are as dedicated to ballet as she is. And the teachers, kids, and parents collectively foster an atmosphere where dancers are more interested in cheering on each other than competing for the spotlight—an atmosphere where everyone belongs and can find collective joy.

Not every group experience will result in feelings of belonging. We have all been part of teams or projects that were unsatisfying or even emotionally unsafe. So let's talk about the ingredients of community and how, as parents, we can seek out places and people who can help our kids experience it.

Tia Kim, the vice president of research at the Committee for Children, defines *belonging* as feeling "valued, accepted, and respected for who you are." Kim told me that "feeling connected to others is a basic human need—people want to feel seen, valued, and cared for by others to feel like they belong."

According to Kim, kids form a sense of belonging when the spaces they inhabit are safe and welcoming. Those spaces can include home, school, neighborhoods, religious organizations, clubs, or teams. Safe and welcoming is the baseline, though. Belonging increases when kids form strong relationships with peers and adults in these spaces. And it is enhanced even more when kids know that they too can contribute to their groups or communities in meaningful ways.

These three prongs of belonging can serve as a useful parenting benchmark:

1. Is your home a safe place? Does your child have at least one additional place where they feel a sense of belonging? This could be school, but it could also be Grandma's house or a neighborhood playgroup.

2. Does your child have strong relationships with both peers and adults—siblings, friends, classmates, parents, teachers, and/or extended family members? How can you support them in strengthening these relationships? The quality of these relationships matters more than the quantity.

3. Are there opportunities for your child to contribute meaningfully in your home and in their other communities? Do

they feel needed—that their community would not be as strong if they were not a part of it?

Needing to Be Needed

A couple of months ago, a bout of food poisoning knocked me flat. It took all my energy to stumble from bed to the bathroom. It was a Sunday night, and my brain ran through what needed to happen around the house. That part of my brain never seems to shut off: feed and walk the dog, make dinner for the kids, clean up from dinner, make sure everyone has finished their homework, start the laundry . . .

I couldn't do any of it—nor could my husband, equally sick beside me—and so my kids did it all. They took out the dog, fed themselves, cleaned up, finished their homework—and got to bed at a decent hour, all while checking in on their poor parents a few times.

Like most kids, my kids complain about chores. But they didn't complain that night. In fact, they almost seemed excited to rise to the challenge. Fred Rogers, per usual, got it right when he wrote, "Whether we're a preschooler or a young teen, a graduating college senior or a retired person, we human beings all want to know that we're acceptable, that our being alive somehow makes a difference in the lives of others."[6]

KJ Dell'Antonia, author of *How to Be a Happier Parent*, once told a story that has stayed with me.[7] After a huge New England snowstorm, a friend's car got stuck going down Dell'Antonia's driveway. She and her four children bundled up and headed out with shovels. After freeing the car once, it slid into a snowbank, and they had to start again as the sun was setting. It was "hard, unpleasant work." Yet after getting the friend safely on her way, one of the children turned to Dell'Antonia and said, "That was fun!"

This story is emblematic of the paradoxes of community and family life. If a child doesn't feel needed, they feel less connected—even if they grumble about those responsibilities. "A kid who has everything done for them begins to see themselves as a job for their parents instead of as a joy or a help," Dell'Antonia told me. This harms kids in at least two ways. It leads to "an artificial sense of their own importance" while also undercutting the valuable role they can play if we let them.

"Everyone is happier when they are part of a larger community," Dell'Antonia went on. "For kids, the family is that first community. When they are part of the day-to-day running of a household, it tells them, *I'm part of the team, and without me, things don't work as well.* They feel like they are a helpful and necessary part of their family." Viewing children as inherently capable changes our approach to interacting with them. "They can do things," she said. "But we mostly don't let them."

My friend Bethany agrees. A mom of three kids under nine, Bethany tells her children, "We all live in the house, so we all have to love it together." Another friend shared that her niece wanted a toy vacuum when she was a preschooler. Instead, her parents got her a small working vacuum for about the same price. "She loved vacuuming right alongside her parents," my friend shared. "I think she could really feel the difference between actually helping and just playing at helping."

In an interview for an NPR article, child psychologist Lauren Silvers talks about how overindulgence can undermine children's role in the family.[8] She defines overindulgence as giving into kids' "whims and desires because you don't want to see them frustrated or uncomfortable, or want to avoid conflict." According to Silvers, parents can tend to do more for their kids than necessary. As a result, she said, "Parents are over-functioning, and then it causes the child to under-function." I need to put that quote on a sticky note on my mirror. Confession: I am a compulsive over-functioner in our home. Sometimes, I feel smug resentment about "all that I do around here for everyone." That's not a dynamic I want to model or pass on. Being a noble martyr doesn't serve anyone well.

Do your kids know how essential they are in your home? Do they feel that sense of purpose and responsibility? Melinda Wenner Moyer, author of *How to Raise Kids Who Aren't A**holes: Science-Based Strategies for Better Parenting—from Tots to Teens*, shared this with me: "There is a strong link between doing things that are good for the whole family and the development of generous behavior. When I ask my kids to help clear the table, I might say, *This is really helping me and dad out, because we have a lot going on. You're making our house look nicer, and you're making it so that we have clean dishes for breakfast tomorrow. So it's really helpful for the entire family.*"

Talking to our kids about their influence is a sign of respect. According to Moyer, it tells them, "You really matter. What you do really affects others. Your actions are powerful and can be used in very, very good ways." And that's pretty awesome, if you ask me.

Belonging Looks Different for Tweens and Teens

We can't talk about awe, belonging, and community without addressing the social dynamics of adolescence, since the urge to belong at this age can both fuel and undermine positive group experiences. Few people know more about that topic than Mitch Prinstein, a professor of psychology and neuroscience at the University of North Carolina, Chapel Hill, and the author of *Popular: The Power of Likability in a Status-Obsessed World*. I spoke to Prinstein on the phone about the importance of belonging for this age group and the role awe can play.

According to Prinstein, an adolescent's desire to feel connected to a peer group has biological and evolutionary roots. A year or so before physical puberty, the brain increases oxytocin receptors, prompting kids to bond more with their peers. This makes sense from an evolutionary standpoint: Joining peer groups that protected each other and worked together was crucial to early humans' survival. Prinstein explained it like this: "Sixty thousand years ago, once you looked like an adult, you had to act like an adult. You were kicked out of the 'house' and had to be autonomous. Today, not so much, but still our brain is making us biologically crave that kind of social interaction so that we feel autonomous—like we're not just being taken care of by our parents anymore."

Peer groups often shuffle and reshuffle during middle and high school and play a role in teens' identity formation. As an adolescent, "you don't want to be part of the group that makes you feel bad about yourself; you want to be part of the group that makes you feel good about yourself," said Prinstein. "You are striving to find people who can be your mirror so you can say, *That's who I am. I'm one of them.*"

This desire to belong to a peer group can be a double-edged sword. Peer groups can be incredibly nourishing, offering enjoyment and acceptance. Such groups can exert positive peer pressure at a time when tweens and teens might be less interested in parents' advice. Teens often seek out clubs or teams that reflect their interests and enjoy that feeling of working toward a shared goal. In other words, such groups offer opportunities to feel collective effervescence. But tweens and teens can also seek out more destructive group experiences. At this age, any group is better than no group. The pull to be with peers who accept them—combined with poor risk assessment and sense of invulnerability—can prime teens to make unhealthy choices. Think about the party that gets out of hand or the criticism or attack of a peer on social media. Recently, the "senior prank" at a local high school took a turn when students began throwing water balloons in the hallway, damaging pieces in the school art show. Were these bad kids? Not at all. The desire to be part of a group holds a powerful, sometimes mystifying sway.

The desire to be part of a group also fuels another social phenomenon: popularity. *Popularity* is a loaded word. It may conjure up unpleasant memories of peers jockeying for position in the high school cafeteria. But understanding this concept can give parents valuable context for what is happening in our kids' brains and with their peers.

According to Prinstein, there are two distinct types of popularity: likability and status. Likability is the first form of popularity that kids experience. "At the age of three, you can go in and ask kids who they like most and least. The popular kids are the ones everyone likes the most," said Prinstein. Children are drawn to peers who treat others with respect, who share and cooperate, and who make others in the group feel good about themselves.

But as children enter middle school, the equation changes. Because of the increase in both oxytocin and dopamine, tweens and teens "become almost addicted to any type of attention from peers," said Prinstein. And unfortunately, one of the fastest ways to get peer attention is to exercise dominance, aggression, and power. Thus enters the second form of popularity: status. Status is not a measure of how well a person is liked. Instead, it reflects a person's visibility, dominance, and influence on the group. (Prinstein likens status-seeking to a primate beating its chest to show dominance.) And that's why the most popular students are sometimes widely disliked by their peers. It can get confusing because your kid may suddenly seek to emulate or be included by the "popular kids"—even if they don't particularly like them.

Here's an important idea to share with all teens: Likeability—not status—predicts positive outcomes decades later, said Prinstein. Unfortunately, this broader vision doesn't reduce the desire to be accepted in a peer group right now.

When Kids Struggle to Fit In

Natalie Bunner knows all about kids' hunger for peer approval. Bunner is the founder/CEO of Thrive Therapy, a pediatric mental health practice in Lafayette, Louisiana. In the teeming sea of social media parenting advice, Bunner consistently offers grounded wisdom. So I reached out to ask her about this topic.

Bunner told me that the kids who come to her office for treatment often struggle to understand "what went wrong" in their efforts to connect with peers. "They want to make friends, to be a part of a group and valued as they are," she said, "but it is hard!"

Bunner has noticed "three consistent elements kids experience in their challenge to belong," and these obstacles are rarely created by the child.

First, children's desire to belong can be overwhelmed by their fear of rejection. Kids who have been rejected before, even at a young age, can form the belief that "belonging may not be a viable option for them" and may become "hypervigilant around rejection, real or perceived."

Second, they may spend time in environments that are "not truly inclusive in the ways that matter." Kids are quick to pick up on signals from adults—signals that, say, reward compliant or high-achieving kids and leave others feeling invisible or less-than.

Finally, kids sometimes have limited opportunities to connect with others based on shared interests or abilities. Bunner told me that parents can think too narrowly in their efforts to help kids connect. For example, parents may push a sport or activity that is "widely accepted in their community" but that does not resonate with their child. Ultimately, this can make a kid feel more displaced.

So how do we help our kids find their people? The good news is that there isn't just one solution, said Bunner. "There are several ways to enrich your child's sense of belonging."

1. Listen carefully to your child. This goes back to radical curiosity. Pay attention to how your child views their social world and brainstorm ways to connect with others. "In this context, your job is to coach, not control," says Bunner. "Confidence grows as they find social strategies that work for them."

2. Give your child an opportunity to try new things. "Abandon the perspective that the only options are standard activities,"

says Bunner. Sometimes our kids need gentle steering to help them find communities that bring out the best in them and give them a sense of belonging—whether it's a chess club, the school newspaper, a coding club, or a band. They also need permission to dabble and shift to new activities when something is not the right fit. Follow your child's curiosities and interests and look for possibilities that match.

3. Prioritize direct connection over virtual belonging. For some kids, connecting online has become a singular, preferred way to engage with others. But Bunner urges parents to help kids seek balance. "Eliminating technology from your child's existence will prove impossible, so reconfigure your perspective about that," she said. "Instead, educate your children. Social media should be a resource, not *the* source for connection."

Learning from Coaches

I really struggled with social connections during middle school. Luckily, high school opened new possibilities. The emotional memories of those four years flow back easily: the adrenaline rush of working late-night deadlines with the school newspaper staff, the thrill of backstage on opening night, and the reverie of singing around the campfire in harmony with my cabinmates. Just last week, a friend from high school texted me an old newspaper clipping about a civics competition from our junior year, and we both agreed it was a life-changing experience.

None of these experiences would have been as awe-inspiring for me without the adults who nurtured the group along: the journalism advisor, the drama director, the camp counselors, and the history teacher. They provided the secret sauce. Clubs, teams, and other group experiences not only expand kids' social nets and help them find belonging, they also give them access to adult mentors who are laser-focused on helping the group progress toward a common goal. Adults in these roles can set the stage for collective effervescence.

Coaching is an art and a science. And, as parents, we all coach our kids. We guide, correct, cheerlead, coax, draw up plays, celebrate wins, teach values, foster family team spirit, and, at the end of the day, tell them to hit the showers. That's why I reached out to a few youth sports coaches. I thought their expertise might be adaptable to our parenting as we work to seek out awe by building community in our homes and neighborhoods. As you read their advice, think about a time from your youth when you felt deeply connected to a group working together on something meaningful. How did adults support this experience? What did they do that increased your joy and belonging? And what do you wish they would have done?

First, meet Bill Tracy. Tracy has spent thirty-two years as a coach, including twenty-three as a head football coach in New Jersey high schools. He loves this work, partly because of the challenge of reaching kids individually while helping shape them into a unified team. And it *is* a challenge. "One of my mentors told me once that if we could get inside the mind of a teenager and figure it all out, we'd be millionaires," said Tracy. "You do your best to be in tune with each kid on your team, with where they are at. And you have to pay attention all the time because they are always telling you something." Remember when your kids were toddlers and everyone told you that, for toddlers, behavior is communication? That doesn't change.

Building a strong community on the field requires really knowing each player. "Knowing your kids is really important," said Tracy. "Set goals with them. See what is on their mind. Wish them good luck on their test today or in their other activities. Connection begins with genuinely caring. My coaches and I want them to know they are valued completely."

While this culture-building takes time, it is what sets the stage for moments of collective effervescence. Tracy told me that "eventually, an 'aha' moment comes when players work in concert with each other and feel that positive energy and culture. They are playing better because of that. You will see teammates cheer on a kid who doesn't play a lot but makes a good play, letting them know they are a key team member—because they are."

Next, meet Mark Semioli, a retired professional soccer player who now coaches youth sports and teaches middle school history in New Jersey. "I have been involved in sports my whole life," he told me. "I've played professionally, I've coached professionally, and now I coach kids. These days, fewer endeavors are *shared* endeavors. With fracturing due to social media and other factors, how often do kids and adults work together in person toward a common purpose?"

When Semioli described how he thinks about forming a "true team," I couldn't help but see it as a metaphor for parenting, as you can see in my bracketed asides.

> First, get your athletes *[kids]* involved in creating the expectations for the team *[the family]*: Who do you want to be? Where do you want to go? Then you need to think about how you are going to help these kids collectively rise to this challenge. They don't need you as a friend; they need you as a coach, a teacher, a guide, and a mentor. If I had to give coaches *[parents]* some advice, I'd say:
>
> ▎ Be clear. Establish a shared purpose and be clear about your expectations.
>
> ▎ Be passionate. Show them you love this work *[family life]*. If you have joy, they will feel it too.
>
> ▎ Be present. When you are there for those two hours of coaching *[afterschool carpools]*, you are nowhere else. You are not looking at your phone. When a kid scores a goal, you are cheering. Pay attention to your weakest players *[your kid who is struggling for XYZ reason this week]*. If you can make your weakest players stronger,

you can find success, because they can find success. That's hard, important work.

About halfway through our conversation, Semioli paused and asked me, "Can I share an unexpected source of awe that occurred during Covid?" Semioli was coaching town soccer, so when schools and other programs shut down, he decided to hold optional, outdoor practices for his team every day that summer—spacing the kids out on the field. "It was a simple come-as-you-want open practice," he said. "We slowly got more and more kids joining in because we were the only thing running."

That fall season, his team didn't lose a single game. "But that wasn't the awe part," he said. "That feeling came from watching these kids dedicate themselves so fully to this sport and to this team. Under difficult circumstances, they decided to commit themselves to something beyond themselves. And they fell in love with it. Our team has since disbanded, but almost all the players have stuck with soccer. That was my awe year."

"I was on a bus with my soccer team coming home from a game. It was a long bus ride, but a little bit into the journey on the way home one of my teammates asked if we could play some music. The sound was turned up and the sun was going down and everyone just started singing. Everyone agreed that it was the best bus ride ever. There was just something there beyond words."—Ava, high schooler

When I spoke to Amy Koehler, a three-season high school athlete who went on to play college basketball, she spoke from a personal and parental perspective. "Sports gave me so much," she told me. "Namely, self-confidence on and off the court, positive body image, and, most of all, the idea of being a team and a leader. I learned the importance of hard work and pushing yourself to be your best for your team's benefit. And I saw how fun, inclusive, and uplifting it is to have a team by your side for joys and losses and the life in between."

Koehler's kids are now young athletes, and she has spent years coaching both her son's and daughter's basketball teams. In the world of youth sports, she has seen many coaches who build positive cultures and a few who foster toxic ones. And of course, she has seen parents on the sidelines engaging in the full spectrum of behavior.

Here's what she wants parents to remember. First, find the fun. "Kids should be playing sports for enjoyment first and foremost, either because they love playing the sport or because they love being with their friends, and ideally both." Second, prioritize equity. "From a very young age, kids can see when coaches favor some players over others. What's our goal? Having fun, learning a sport, getting better, being a team—all those goals are fostered when everyone plays, is involved, and feels included. Winning is fun, but you can have a losing season and still achieve every one of those goals." Finally, make sure you are modeling inclusive, kind behavior. "Parents are the glue," said Koehler. "Families need to surround the team with positivity."

In fact, all the coaches I spoke with named parents' behavior and how it could strengthen or damage the team experience. Semioli told me, "Parents directly affect the experience of their kids. If parents share their frustrations with coaches in front of their kid or do not seem to enjoy the game, that takes away from a player's feelings of awe."

Tracy offered this reflection: "It can be tricky to be a parent in the stands because it's your child, and you are passionate about your child. But there's only a small window in your lives together where you can enjoy watching your child play. Do your best to enjoy it. Only about 5 percent of high school athletes play varsity sports in college, and far less than that go on to play in the pros. So just enjoy the game for what it is right now, at this moment."

Creative Coaching: Pete's Story

Five years ago, Pete Munene founded the Harambee Sports Club—a nonprofit that provides programs to support and connect diverse youth and their communities in the Twin Cities of Minnesota. Munene believes that youth sports can be transformational if coaches are intentional about social and emotional learning. Sometimes, that means thinking creatively. Take the Houseplant Project. Munene got his first plant when he was nine years old. "It was important to me. It was something I could take care of; it was lovely, and it was mine," he said. A few years ago, he thought to himself, *What if I could provide that feeling for my players? I have access to these kids, and I have access to plants, so why not?* After all, winters are long in Minnesota—and a little green can help.

Munene began to propagate his own plants, but he also asked the community for help. People quickly signed up to donate—and when they dropped off plants, they also shared stories. One person brought in a set of plants that were offshoots of a houseplant his grandmother had tended. Munene was surprised by how excited people were to give plants—and how excited kids were to receive them: "Do these plants make kids better soccer players?" he said. "Does it matter? What we do know is that this program has made the children's community a little bit bigger and their homes a little bit brighter."

Belonging and the Performing Arts

I wasn't much of an athlete growing up, but I loved theater: going to the shows, listening to cast recordings, taking drama classes, and working backstage on high school productions. When I became a teacher, I often orchestrated small classroom productions. Sometimes I noticed that quieter students could don, say, a silly hat and suddenly project a new persona. As one theater producer told me, "Broadway stages are full of introverts."

Putting on a play is a truly collective experience: Everyone needs to show up for the show to go on. That feeling when the audience claps and cheers as you bow? Magical. Being in the audience this winter when my daughter took a bow during the curtain call for *The Diary of Anne Frank*? Pure wonder.

New Victory Theater in New York City is a global leader in arts education. Their programs aim to bring "kids to the arts and the arts to kids." I spoke with Dennie Palmer Wolf, a leading arts researcher who has studied New Victory's programs, and Lindsey Buller Maliekel, the theater's vice president for education and public engagement.

Watching theater is a "shared emotional experience," said Maliekel. "The audience is feeling things collectively." She and her team love watching kids' faces when they come to a show. "We sometimes talk about it as *wide eyes*—like, *oh, they've got really wide eyes*—which is our way of naming the moment when a world opened up that was not present in the room when they arrived."

New Victory partnered with the research firm WolfBrown to investigate the impact of performing arts on kids. For this, New Victory went into public elementary and middle schools that were devoid of arts experiences. "They had no arts teachers; they had no arts clubs," said Maliekel. According to New Victory's Impact Research Report, providing students with access to and engagement with the performing arts has four measurable outcomes:[9]

1. It "cultivates an enduring love of performing arts."

2. It "expands perspectives and interpersonal skills that strengthen teamwork."

3. It "inspires creative thinking, which encourages innovation and problem-solving."

4. It "nurtures hope and improves self-confidence, which fosters optimism and resilience."

The researchers were surprised by the finding that participation in performing arts "gave students hope." After participating for just one year in New Victory's school arts program, elementary-age children's "future orientation" scores increased by over 10 percent. That means more students responded affirmatively to survey questions such as "I will graduate from high school." In contrast, during that same period, the control group saw a 5 percent decrease in their future orientation scores.

Maliekel described a phenomenon she and Wolf would repeatedly experience when they walked into New York City public school classrooms. "There was this moment when a group of young people were able to imagine themselves and each other differently. That happened over and over again, so much that it appears in the research." In essence, they observed kids saying, "I can imagine a world that is better than the one I'm living in. I can imagine a future for myself that is different from the one I live in now."

Wolf shared a memory from an elementary school visit. New Victory had been working with students for several months, and that day, the kids were learning the circus art of plate spinning. "The teaching artists demonstrated it, and the kids were quite convinced they could not do it," said Wolf. "But he broke it down in such a way that they could." Soon, she watched a trio of boys, who were not particular friends, work together. "They became so captivated by the fact that the plate went up, that it stayed there, and that the least likely of them was capable of doing this feat. For a micro moment, all three of them—spinner and spin watchers—transformed."

Maliekel also witnessed this. "The young people's capacity to do something they thought was impossible was part of the transformation and part of the awe. Their reactions said, *What, this is me? Wait, this is him? Could never be!* But it was."

These performance experiences—like so many moments of everyday awe—add up over time, strengthening kids' sense of hope, joy, and belonging.

"My theater troupe worked hard for months to perform a fifteen-minute cut of a musical at the Junior Theater Festival, a musical theater festival in Atlanta, Georgia. We performed *James and the Giant Peach*, and I got to play the role of James. When our director told us we won, we felt incredible. I was so proud and amazed that all our hard work paid off in this extraordinary way. Some of us had tears of joy. Because we won, we got to perform our cut in front of almost seven thousand people. Backstage before our performance, I felt anxious, but as soon as the announcer called our theater's name and the crowd cheered, I was pumped up. Being on stage in front of all those people feels hard to explain. It was mind-blowing. It was really cool. Because the lights were so bright, it was hard to see the audience, but you could really *hear* them. The sound of seven thousand people clapping and cheering for my friends made me feel so proud. It was an honor to be performing the wonderful show we all worked so hard to create. The adrenaline I felt afterwards had me shaking! That whole experience is now one of my core memories."
—Luna Faye, age 12

Rituals, Routines, and Rich Connections

Let's switch gears and talk about something else that creates belonging: rituals and routines. In surveys, adults report feeling awe during collective rituals such as weddings, graduations, and religious ceremonies. However, research shows that even smaller rituals can foster connection—like family dinners.

Dinners at my house can be messy, and I'm not just talking about the countertops. It is hard to coordinate schedules, pull kids away from homework/hobbies/books/sports/screens, put away my own work, and figure out what to cook that the majority of the family will eat. But most nights, all of us are together in the same room, eating something, at dinner-ish time.

When I spoke to Robert Waldinger (you'll remember his name from the introduction), who directs the Harvard Study of Adult Development, about the human happiness study's top findings for parents, he mentioned family dinners. Eating together is a ritual; family rituals and routines are protective, especially as children grow into adolescents and seek more independence.

As Waldinger and Schulz write in *The Good Life*, "Teens need you. Some teens will show this by being clingy, but others may insist they don't need anyone. Of course, they do. In fact, a teen's relationships with adults may be more crucial than at any other time in life. Research tells us that there are advantages for adolescents who become more autonomous while still remaining connected to their parents."[10]

Autonomy *and* connection. That's a tricky dance, especially as kids get older, but sometimes the simplest tools are the most useful. Research shows that regular family dinners correlate with higher grade-point averages, greater self-confidence, and lower rates of substance abuse and depression.[11] If evening meals just don't work in your home, perhaps you can aim for breakfast or a regular family movie night or game night. The point is predictable togetherness.

Don't be surprised if teens start resisting family activities and routines, though. As Waldinger told me, "Teenagers are classically ambivalent. They want to be independent and mature, and they want to stay a little kid." In this turbulence, teens need the comfort and connective tissue provided by family traditions. "Your child might signal, *I don't need my family, to heck with all of you*, and at the same time go along grudgingly and be reassured by the structure," Waldinger says. "It doesn't mean we make our teens do everything. We pick our battles, but some structure really matters. For most kids, it's reassuring that structure stays while they're going through a tumultuous time."

We can also throw a blanket of belonging around children who are not our own. Can you name at least one adult from your childhood, a person other than a parent, who wrapped you up with warmth? In high school, my friends and I would travel as a pack to different houses to study and socialize. We gathered at some homes more than others, but it was never about the size of the house. We gravitated to places where the adults made us feel welcome. That's why we spent so many evenings at the Tanner home. Jon's mom seemed to genuinely enjoy a bunch of gangly teenagers taking over the family room and raiding the pantry. Her face would light up with delight when we barged in unannounced (and since this was before personal devices, it was almost always unannounced). Spaces hold emotional memories. The Tanner home, in my memory, is pure warmth.

A Final Thought

If belonging feels awesome, then exclusion feels awful. All of our kids will experience both as they grow up, though hopefully the balance is tipped toward the former.

I don't know where things are landing in your home right now. School may be a struggle. Your kid might be facing loneliness or social anxiety. Perhaps they are still hunting for that club or activity that speaks to them. Maybe you've moved recently. Or you've switched schools and your kid is still trying to figure out how they fit in. There's so much we can't control, but we can do our best to give our kids a safe place to land.

I'll end this chapter with a story about that.

January can be a tough month to have a birthday as a kid—but even more so in 2021 in frozen New England. Covid cases were spiking, and with no outings, playdates, or parties in the pandemic forecast, we had a pretty dejected six-year-old at home. When I suggested we splurge on a special cake, he responded: "I want a winter woodland animals scene with a pond and with vines wrapped around a red number-seven candle."

While I was still processing the request, his nine-year-old sister piped up: "Oh, I can totally do that for you." And she did, with the support of YouTube, fondant, food coloring, and a $5 tube of plastic animal figurines.

A week later, my son reminded me that his sister's half-birthday was approaching. Listen, we are *not* a celebrate-half-birthdays kind of family. "Please, please, please can I decorate a cake?" he begged. That's how we found ourselves lighting half a candle on an ocean cake, covered with gobs of blue icing and Swedish fish.

"Did you know there is a holiday every single day?" my kids remarked while eating this bright blue cake. "It's not just Halloween and Valentine's Day and stuff. There's National Puppy Day in March, and January 31 is National Hot Chocolate Day. We looked it up on Google."

So on the last day of January, we sipped hot chocolates with mountains of mini marshmallows. It was a cold afternoon, and we likely would have been drinking cocoa anyway. But this wasn't just a snack; it was a celebration.

On February 2, the kids got up early to watch the Groundhog Day broadcast from Punxsutawney, Pennsylvania. We watched men in top hats pull out the rodent and reveal the verdict: six more weeks of winter. Then the Master of Ceremonies opined, "It has felt like at times we're all living the same day over and over again. But Groundhog Day also shows us that the monotony ends. The cycle will be broken." And that's how I found myself tearing up in my PJs at 7:26 a.m. on a Tuesday.

That same afternoon, my kids started a list of February holidays. Our fridge calendar, which for months had been empty of anything beyond Zoom piano lessons, began to fill with Highly Important Events: National Bubble Gum Day (2/5), National Pizza Day (2/9), National Pancake Day (2/16), Random Act of Kindness Day (2/17), National Cherry Pie Day (2/20), National Walking Your Dog Day (2/22), National Clam Chowder Day (2/25), International Polar Bear Day (2/27).

"Did you know this Saturday is National Eat Ice Cream for Breakfast Day?" my brother texted when he heard about my kids' efforts to celebrate absolutely everything. That vision sustained my son for *days*. Every morning, he would say, "Don't forget, we get to eat ICE CREAM for breakfast on Saturday." In a year marked with macro-drama and yet tedious monotony, these micro-celebrations brought pockets of wonder to our family life.

That's why I said yes to all the winter "holidays." That's why on February 14, in addition to eating pink pancakes for Valentine's Day, we put on our coats to join the Audubon Society's Great Backyard Bird Count.

"Did you hear that? What makes that call?"

"There's one! Take a picture! Look it up—it's gray and white and orange!"

"That's a hawk up there! It's soaring!"

In forty-five minutes, we submitted sightings of tufted titmouses, a Cooper's hawk, a downy woodpecker, black-capped chickadees, and a northern cardinal.

"I really like birds, Mom," my newly-seven-year-old said, slipping his hand into my coat pocket. "Can we celebrate this holiday every year?"

Yes, of course. But first and foremost, we can celebrate that we belong to each other, every single day.

5 Wonderful Ways to Help Kids Experience Belonging

1. Get to Know Your Neighbors. Do your kids know the names of at least some of your neighbors? Building a community can start on your block or in your apartment building. As a family, look for simple ways to be neighborly—like taking out the trash bins of an elderly neighbor, dropping off kid-made holiday cards, or taking a plate of cookies to the family who just moved in.

2. Attend a Community Celebration. Does your city or town have any rituals that your family can join—like a Memorial Day parade, carnival, holiday stroll, 5K, or sporting event? These types of experiences can help kids feel more connected to the place they live.

3. Connect with the School. One of the best predictors of children's overall well-being is school connectedness. Kids who feel safe and welcome at school do better on almost every measurable outcome. And children feel more connected when their parents are connected—from attending back-to-school night to being in communication with their children's teachers.

4. Tell Family Stories. A study found that children who hear stories about how family members overcame obstacles are more resilient in the face of challenges.[12] Strong family narratives are protective, reminding kids that they belong to something larger than themselves. And as kids learn about how other people navigate life's ups and downs, they develop multiple mental blueprints for how to do this themselves.

5. Sync Up. Collective effervescence happens when a group works in harmony toward a common goal. Encourage your kid to test out groups, activities, teams, or clubs that match their interests, so that they can meet peers with similar interests. Not every group will be a good fit, and that's okay. Keep trying.

10 Awe-Inspiring Picture Books About Belonging and Community

Our Table **by Peter H. Reynolds.** Violet's family is not as connected as it used to be due to schedules and distractions. She misses the way they used to gather at the table. So she decides to do something about it. This book reads like a modern-day magical fable.

Finding Winnie: The True Story of the World's Most Famous Bear **by Lindsay Mattick and Sophie Blackall.** Discover the power of family stories as author Lindsay Mattick shares one of her own family stories—about the great-grandfather for whom her son is named and the real bear who became the beloved Winnie-the-Pooh. Don't skip the album at the back with the author's real family photos and artifacts.

Apart, Together: A Book About Transformation **by Linda Booth Sweeney and Ariel Rutland.** Apart, yellow is yellow and blue is blue—but together, they are green. Soap and water, together, make bubbles. This book is a lovely way to explore ways that our differences make us stronger, together.

Goal! **by Mina Javaherbin and A. G. Ford.** On the streets of a South African township, a group of enthusiastic young soccer players confront bullies and celebrate the unifying power of soccer.

ZooZical **by Judy Sierra and Marc Brown.** Winter doldrums have overtaken the zoo's animals, and so they decide to put on a show. A grand musical—er, ZooZical—allows every animal to participate in a mood-lifting performance.

Stone Soup **by Jon J. Muth.** This book is a refreshing retelling of an old story. Three monks arrive in a Chinese mountain village that has become selfish and distrustful. The clever monks gently trick them into remembering the joy that comes from true community.

Ada's Violin: The Story of the Recycled Orchestra of Paraguay **by Susan Hood and Sally Wern Comport.** Ada wants to play the violin, but that seems like an impossibility until a music teacher finds a way to create instruments out of recycled trash. Based on the true story of the Recycled Orchestra of Paraguay.

Change Sings: A Children's Anthem **by Amanda Gorman and Loren Long.** In poet Amanda Gorman's first picture book, a young girl and her guitar gather a diverse band of child musicians, who together figure out how to change their community in small and big ways.

Packs: Strength in Numbers **by Hannah Salyer.** Animals of all kinds live in groups (or pods, packs, herds, and flocks). That includes humans. This nonfiction book celebrates how animals rely on each other to survive and thrive.

All of Us **by Kathryn Erskine and Alexandra Boiger.** This simple, lovely book celebrates moving from me to we, from a global perspective. The illustrations are gorgeous and inclusive.

CHAPTER SIX

THE WONDER OF THE CIRCLE OF LIFE

Life's beauty is inseparable from its fragility.
—*Dr. Susan David*

Pause and imagine these faces:

A four-year-old staring at a butterfly perched on their finger.
An eight-year-old snuggling the family's new puppy.
A twelve-year-old holding their one-week-old baby cousin for the first time.
A seventeen-year-old camp counselor bending down to help a preschooler who has fallen.

In my parenting workshops, I sometimes joke that if you have a moody adolescent, try handing them a baby or a puppy and see how their face brightens up. When my kids are reluctant to get up in the morning, I'll send the dog in to jump on their beds and lick their faces. They are far less likely to yell at Cupid than at me.

It's so easy to see how experiences with babies—in both human and animal form—can trigger awe in our kids. Their fragility evokes our instinct to care and protect, to pause and pay attention.

This chapter is all about the wonder of beginnings—and also of endings. There is no birth without death. All of life is wondrous, and there is something compelling about encountering both ends of it.

Dacher Keltner discovered in his research that people are awestruck by the "cycle of life and death." As he told one interviewer, "People around the world find it awe-inspiring when life emerges and when it goes."[1]

Living in the Moment

Strangers' faces often light up when I'm out on a walk. But they're not smiling at me; they're delighted by my fluffy dog. In an interview with NPR, Nancy Gee, director of the Center for Human-Animal Interaction at Virginia Commonwealth University, noted that interacting with dogs—even strangers' dogs—can affect body chemistry. After spending a few minutes with a dog, most people experience a reduction in the stress hormone cortisol and an uptick in the "feel-good" hormone oxytocin. Gee said, "I think it is safe to say that animals are beneficial to our mental and physical health."[2]

But why? Megan Mueller, an associate professor of veterinary medicine at Tufts University, told NPR that dogs prompt us to experience the world more like they do: "Animals, and dogs in particular, live in the moment. They're experiencing their environment with wonder and awe all the time, and they're not bringing up what happened to them earlier in the day or what they're thinking about in the future. They're there right now."[3] According to Mueller, watching dogs pay attention to their environment can prompt us to pay more attention too. "They sort of pull you out of your phone and into whatever environment that you're in."

Perhaps this is part of why holding a baby or watching a butterfly emerge from a chrysalis can prompt awe: For a baby or a butterfly, there is only *now*. This moment. That's something we and our older kids can struggle to feel. When I taught middle and high school, I could see the challenge of students being "present" when class started—not with their bodies, but with their minds.

"How many of you are in the past or the future right now?" I once asked. "Are you thinking about that conversation you had before school? Or worrying about the quiz in your next class?" Every hand went up. Sometimes, I'd have students take one minute and just jot down everything swirling around in their brains. Sometimes, I would sound a chime and ask them to listen until the sound dissipated. Take a deep breath. Try to be in the moment.

My daughter's favorite day of the week is Tuesday, because that's when middle schoolers spend an hour volunteering in a preschool classroom. Three-year-olds aren't thinking about essay deadlines or rehearsal schedules or science tests. They don't worry about acne or Instagram. One Tuesday, a little girl grabbed my daughter's hand and announced, "You are so big! Can you read me a story? I will sit here on your lap, and you can read and read."

Sam, a high school junior in Massachusetts, has also discovered something wonderful while working with preschoolers. His public high school is home to the Child Lab—a preschool that is essentially run by students under the tutelage of the Lab's director. Students study child development and design lessons and activities. Sam told me that working in the Child Lab has been one of the best experiences of his high school career. He said, "When I am in the middle of a long school day, stepping back and revisiting the joys of childhood is a great way to ground myself. I forget calculus and Shakespeare for dinosaurs and simple machines. Getting to be a positive influence on these kids' lives is a great feeling, especially since I know how amazing role models made me feel in my formative years."

A common thread from these studies and stories is this: When we slow down and savor the moment, we make room for awe to enter. For our older kids especially, spending time with little ones and animals can help them savor the *now*.

"I was in the hospital the day after my cousin gave birth. When I finally held her baby, it was love at first sight. I knew that it was my job to protect her and treat her like the little sister I never got to have."
—Alejandra, middle schooler

"I felt awe when I went up to Maine with my family to pick out a puppy we would soon take home. As we walked into the building, a storm of golden retriever puppies greeted us eagerly, tails wagging and ears flapping. We soon got to hold each of the puppies, and as my arms wrapped around one of the little creatures, my heart filled. The adorable puppy was looking up at me with small, curious eyes, full of innocence and happiness. He squirmed in my arms for a minute or two, but soon settled down so I could pet his soft fur."
—Grace, middle schooler

Cosmic Questions

Young kids are fascinated with birth and death. Just think about the wonder in your child's eyes when you recount a story from their newborn days. To many parents' consternation, though, children can become somewhat obsessed with death. It is, after all, one of life's biggest questions. As we watched the sun go down after a long day at the beach one summer, my then-three-year-old daughter turned to me and asked, "Mommy, where does the sun go at night? Does it fall into the ocean? Does it turn into the moon? Does it *die*?"

Developmentally, preschoolers usually don't understand that death is permanent and irreversible. But they are curious about it and often sense that it's a tricky topic for adults. School-age children start to develop a more realistic understanding of death. They may have a lot of questions and even develop fears about their own death or the deaths of loved ones. The older kids get, the more experience they inevitably have with loss. And this will lead to new questions and emotions.

In Keltner's book *Awe*, some of the most moving passages are reflections on the death of his brother. In a 2023 interview with *Big Think*, Keltner shared that he receives daily emails about that section of the book, with people writing things like, "I just lost my brother. I lost my child. I lost my mom." Death opens the mind to wonder and awe, said Keltner. "What is this life we are given about? What happens when people die? How are those people still with us? Those are perennial questions. They're essential, and awe is a great catalyst for growth—as I discovered thankfully."[4]

A Tale of Two Butterflies

Let me tell you a story about kids and death.

One June afternoon, I sent my tantruming then-six-year-old to his room and sent myself to mine. We were having a *day*. After taking a few deep breaths, I went and found him hiding under his stuffed animals. "You've got a lot of mad inside you," I said.

"I'm mad because I am sad! Duh!" he responded, his voice muffled.

"Sad?"

"*You* know—because something is dead that should be alive!"

The day before, he had rescued a caterpillar from the window ledge. My creature-loving kid ran outside to collect leaves and carefully placed them in a mason jar. He then spent much of the evening gazing at his new pet. But the next morning, his sister noticed the caterpillar was dead. I cleaned out the jar while doing the breakfast dishes.

Now here we were, six hours later. My son's anger melted into sobs once he named the pain. I don't suppose he felt anything remotely close to awe at that moment. But his simple statement, "I'm mad because I'm sad," was nothing short of an epiphany. I had been agitated all week, and my outsized reaction to my son's tantrums also had roots in grief.

Father's Day was approaching, and I was missing my dad. Someone was dead who should be alive. He should have had a chance to meet his grandkids. Once I paused long enough to name the sadness, relief flooded in.

After the death of that caterpillar, we bought a butterfly kit. At the appointed time, all the butterflies emerged from their chrysalises except one—this last creature poked out a single wing, and then stopped. At my son's suggestion, we Googled "butterfly is having a hard time getting out of chrysalis." After careful researching, we resolved to help our friend along by making a tiny opening in the shell. Out popped a beautiful butterfly, with only one wing and three legs. It could not stand. As the other butterflies drank from the sugar-water sponge, it lay on its side, twitching.

The kids debated whether we should just raise this butterfly in a jar. "No. It needs to be outside," my son insisted. "That's where butterflies belong. It's what they know." His sister built a nest of maple leaves and purple flowers in the front yard and then gently laid the fragile creature within. "I think we should name her Faith," she said, "because we believed in her." When it was clear our butterfly was dead, my kids detached the single wing and set it on our mantel. "It's so sad, and it's so beautiful," my son said.

Our instinct is often to want to shield kids from discussions of sickness, death, and sadness. But sickness and death are part of life. Sadness holds hands with joy. If we feel awe when we encounter the vast and the mysterious, then beginnings and endings offer opportunities for our children to experience this emotion. After all, a core emotional lesson for kids is realizing that we can feel more than one thing at once. We can be happy and sad, excited and scared, worried and hopeful.

A few years ago, I published a picture book about emotions called *You Have Feelings All the Time*. One of the pages is about mixed feelings:

> Feelings also come in twos.
> You're happy AND you're sad.

You're glad that mom is coming home,
but when grandma leaves, you're mad.

When I first read the book to preschoolers, I was amazed by how well four- and five-year-olds were able to articulate their own moments of mixed feelings. One child talked about releasing a helium balloon: It felt so exciting to watch it fly high, but then he was so sad it was gone.

A good word to describe these connected feelings is *poignancy*. It's that feeling we have when our child walks across the stage at graduation: pride at their accomplishment but perhaps melancholy knowing that this stage of their life (and ours) is ending. I remember becoming tearful before my youngest's sixth birthday because 1) I love watching my kids grow and 2) I was so sad that I would never have a five-year-old again. As a teacher, I felt this at the end of each school year: excited for summer, proud of my students' growth, but sad that our time together was ending. Poignancy, like awe, is a rich emotion. And poignancy can signal that we're in a moment ripe for finding awe: We can feel awe in the letting go, in marveling how far our kids have come, and acknowledging that our care helped get them there. We can miss what was while looking with wonder toward all our kids might be in the future.

The Wisdom of Elders

Last fall, an eighth grader at The Rashi School in Dedham, Massachusetts, asked me this question: "In your research, have you figured out why kids are more connected to their elders in some cultures than in others?"

I was walking with a group of students from the school to a senior living center. It was only a three-minute walk, by design. Several years ago, Rashi—a preK–8 Jewish day school—built its new campus across the street from a large senior living center to "foster a community where people live and learn across generations." From preschool through middle school, Rashi students build relationships with the residents at NewBridge on the Charles. The interactions between generations can be planned or informal, like the group of residents I saw who stopped to wave at preschoolers on the playground.

"Do you think kids and older adults should be more connected?" I replied to my walking companion.

"Absolutely," said the middle schooler. "They've lived through so much. We have a lot to learn from them."

On this autumn day, the eighth graders were making their weekly visit to the memory unit. One student emphasized that she calls it a *visit*, not *service*, because "I love my resident! It's so fun to go visit her." Rashi trains their oldest students on best practices for interacting with adults with advanced dementia. The kids know the residents probably won't remember them from week to week. And yet, I saw nothing but smiles from the residents and the students as we walked into the room. They began working together on a simple art project. I sat next to a student who chatted effortlessly with her senior buddy. Here's a snippet of their conversation:

> Resident: "What does your mom do?"
> Student: "She's a teacher."
> Resident: "I was a teacher!"
> Student: "I bet you were a great teacher."
> Resident: "I love your bracelet."
> Student: "Thank you so much! I got it for my birthday."
> Resident: "It is beautiful. You are beautiful. Just beautiful."

As I walked around the room, I was struck by the students' genuine interest—how they leaned forward, listened, and asked questions. One boy sat with a quiet man, gently guiding his hand as he colored. Another student introduced me to a resident who had just turned 102, saying, "Can you imagine how much she's seen?"

As we prepared to leave, I talked to one of the center's staff members. "These visits make such a difference," he said. "The residents are happier on Fridays after the students come. They even eat better. We all feel how the tone shifts."

Rabbi Sharon Clevenger works at The Rashi School. She describes the partnership with NewBridge as a relationship of equals: "The seniors come in and help our kids, and we go over and entertain and help the seniors. We bring youth, and they bring age. We bring curiosity; they bring curiosity coupled with wisdom." The partnership also brings kids face-to-face with something else: death. Residents will pass away, and that is something adults and kids talk about together.

Rabbi Clevenger understands why many parents feel reluctant to talk with kids about death. Still, she says we need to find ways to normalize these conversations. "To shield children entirely from death and the dying process—and even the aging process—is doing them a disservice," she told me. "Everybody dies. Death is just a bookend of life. And to let that be something that's secret? Unspoken things become more frightening to children, giving them a power that they don't have to have. When I think about death, I think about death as a reminder to us that we need to live our best lives."

Rabbi Clevenger's words resonated with my experience. When I was growing up, my maternal grandparents lived with us, and Grandma was largely immobile because of advanced osteoporosis. Some of my earliest memories include lounging on the side of her large armchair while my mom fixed her hair, "helping" the physical therapist who came to our home each week, and playing finger games like "Where Is Thumbkin?" with Grandma. She died in our home, when I was six. After that, I started spending more and more time with Grandpa, who at that point was ninety-five. We liked each other's company. He was a retired farmer who kept up our garden. I helped him plant peas and thin irises. He made me Grandma's cookies but often overcooked them or put in too much salt. I ate them anyway. When he was ninety-eight, he fell from a stepstool. He wanted to die at home, not in a hospital. A few days later, family surrounded Grandpa's bed as he slipped into a deep sleep from which he would never wake.

I suppose these early experiences with aging and death are what made me uncommonly comfortable with the elderly as an adolescent and a young adult. Our neighborhood was adjacent to a retirement community and many of those residents were also in our church congregation. My mom was an organist, so she was on call for every funeral. I was often sent to deliver cookies or a meal to someone who was recovering from an illness. One of these deliveries led to a friendship with a couple in their late eighties. Lenora told me stories about teaching school in the 1920s and taught me how to make silk roses. When I left for college, I regularly received cards from Lenora—written out by her husband, Arthur, because her handwriting had become too shaky.

Lynda Doctoroff Bussgang is director of volunteer, youth, and community engagement for Hebrew SeniorLife, an organization that runs six senior campuses including the one that Rashi students visit. Her background is in moral development, and she is fascinated by "the concept of passing along experiences and wisdom from generation to generation." For that to happen, she told me, you first need to "bring young people into contact with the older generation." When she works with partnering organizations, she makes it clear that "spending time with seniors is not a service project—it's not a box to check off." Instead, it's a chance to foster connection and relationships.

According to a study by the Stanford Center on Longevity, older adults may be "just the resource children need." The researchers note that older adults have wisdom and complex problem-solving and emotional skills from experience. They conclude, "Older adults are exceptionally suited to meet [the needs of youth] in part because they welcome meaningful, productive activity and engagement. They seek—and need—purpose in their lives."[5]

Rashi and Hebrew SeniorLife are just two of many organizations to get creative about connecting the generations. In Swampscott, Massachusetts, the high school and the senior center share a building.[6] The previous senior center and high school were both aging, so this town of around 15,000 people chose to build a multigenerational space to replace both—a cost-effective decision that has had wonderful ripple effects. The school and the senior center have separate entrances but share common spaces such as the cafeteria, fitness center, and computer labs. Seniors can get tech support from students, and students can drop by the senior center to learn how to knit or to conduct an interview for history class. And in western Massachusetts, you'll find a planned intergenerational community designed to support foster children.[7] Treehouse at Easthampton Meadow offers housing to people ages fifty-five and up and to families who are caring for children from the public foster care system. The idea is to surround these families—and these vulnerable children—with a village of support. These kids get a whole community of foster grandparents to love on them.

"My grandpa is one of those people who always has a new story to tell and if not, he'll just retell his favorite ones. One night after dinner, someone asked him about his favorite childhood memory. He said it was when World War II ended, and then he told the story as if it were yesterday. He was on the Swan Boats in Boston with his friends, and a large group of people were listening to the radio. An announcement came on saying that the war had just ended. People ran into the streets cheering and crying and hugging each other. There were so many people that it took my grandpa and his friends an hour to get home to South Boston by trolley car. I could tell that my grandpa loved that memory the most because he had tears in his eyes when he finished telling us about it."—Keira, high schooler

These initiatives fill me with awe and give me hope. And they make me ask how we can be more intentional about linking the generations. I'll admit that my own kids are not as connected to older adults as I was growing up, and I'm sad about that. Perhaps reading this will give you a spark of wonder and help you get creative in finding ways to link generations in your family or community.

Helping Kids Navigate Loss

While writing this chapter, I've been thinking about Rabbi Clevenger's comment, "To shield children entirely from death and the dying process—and even the aging process—is doing them a disservice." I've also been thinking about how, in my own multigenerational household, my grandparents aged and died at home. These things were never hidden. All this has led me to two questions: How do we help our kids through loss? And how do we help them find awe in community and kindness amid the pain? Acknowledging that there can be awe at the bookends of life does not mitigate the need to help kids process their grief.

For this one, I'm going back to Mister Rogers.

Sometimes, I feel like Fred Rogers helped raise me. I watched *Mister Rogers' Neighborhood* as a child—waving goodbye and sometimes kissing the TV screen. As an adult, I have used his approach to working with children to cultivate my own. When I was working on an article about him for PBS, a friend reached out to share how Mister Rogers offered her a hand in the darkness during a traumatic childhood: "I can't even read his name without tearing up. During those rough years, *Sesame Street* taught me to read, and Mister Rogers taught me to hope."

Angela Santomero, the creator of *Neighborhood* companion show *Daniel Tiger's Neighborhood*, told me that Rogers taught adults how to talk to kids in an "honest, open, genuine, and respectful way." Rogers approached his conversations with kids with "fearless authenticity," she said, including discussions about life and death.

In December 2023, twelve-year-old Alice lost her friend Cooper. Her poetic tribute to him captures the truth that your sadness means "you really loved that person and you really miss them."

Dear Cooper

Hey Cooper, with the good hair
I'm sad because you're not here anymore
And there are so many things left to say
So, I'll tell you now of my thankfulness

Dear Cooper, did you know your smile
Made everyone smile, too? I'm so thankful.
You made me laugh with your laugh.

Dear Cooper, did you know that
Your screams on roller coasters and waterslides
Showed the whole world your happiness?

Dear Cooper, did you know I *never*
Beat you at Super Smash Brothers?
But now I know how to beat my sister.

Dear Cooper, I've heard Christmas in Heaven is amazing.
I really hope so, because the lights on my tree
Dimmed when you left.

Dear Cooper, did you know how much my heart hurts?
But, I'm so thankful because
It means I got to love you.

As part of every show, Mister Rogers fed his pet fish. One day, he arrived at the set and found a dead goldfish in the aquarium. Rather than replacing the fish without informing his TV audience, he decided to use this moment to talk to his young viewers about death and to share childhood memories about how he felt when his dog died. Santomero said this choice reflects one of Rogers's guiding principles: What is mentionable is manageable. Rogers once said, "Anything that's human is mentionable, and anything that's mentionable can be more manageable.... When we can talk about our feelings, they become less overwhelming, less upsetting, and less scary. The people we trust with that important talk can help us know that we're not alone and that our feelings are natural and normal."[8]

Another wise voice on kids and grief is Hope Edelman. Edelman's mother died when she was seventeen, and she has since turned that loss into something of a vocation, writing books about bereavement, including *The AfterGrief: Finding Your Way Along the Long Arc of Loss.*

Every family wrestles with grief at some point. That grief might be fresh: the death of a family member, a divorce, the loss of a friend, or a new health diagnosis. Or it may be the "long arc": missing a loved one all over again as we experience milestones without them. Think about how an eighth grader who loses her mother might feel that loss anew before her first high school dance, when she gets her driver's license, and when she graduates.

Grief can feel particularly acute during the holidays. Edelman taught me the phrase *grief spike*—an intensity of emotion that hits us suddenly during holidays, milestones, or anniversaries. These times remind us of who's not there to celebrate with us. Edelman says that one of the best things parents can do for grieving kids is to make space for their relationships with the deceased to continue. She told me: "One of the hardest things for a child, especially over time, is to lose someone and then not be able to talk about that person anymore. When the child is silenced, then they're left trying to have a relationship with that person by themselves. Kids will talk pretty openly about people who've died if we create the space for them to do that." When we encourage kids to share their memories, it "helps cement their connection to the person who's no longer here."

Tangible activities can also help kids stay connected after loss. This might look like cooking a grandparent's special recipe, lighting a candle in someone's memory, or telling stories about a loved one around the holiday table. It may also look like carrying on one of their favorite traditions or creating a new tradition in their honor. Edelman said, "Rituals give kids a feeling that they belong to something larger than themselves."

I lost my dad a couple of years before my first child was born. When I have a grief spike of missing him, one way I work through those feelings is by telling my kids a Grandpa Jim story. Over the years, they have heard about the beautiful ways they are like him—in their curiosity, love of chocolate, and fascination with gadgets and mythology. These stories give me an excuse to remember him, to say his name, and to help my children feel connected to a grandfather they never met.

As we help our kids navigate loss, it's important to remember that they process grief differently than we do as adults. A lot depends on a kid's age and temperament. Very young children, for example, may experience the loss as a change in their routine (*I used to visit Grandma on Sunday, and now we don't do that*). As Edelman told me, younger children live very much in the present. They often "only dip into grief very briefly, and then they back away." The term for that is *grief dosing*. A young child may have a short, intense outburst and then run off to play. But that doesn't mean they are not grieving, said Edelman. "It just means that they can only handle grief in very small doses." Teenagers already experience emotional intensity as part of their development, so grief can accentuate their emotions: Anger may grow stronger, and anxiety may grow deeper. Some teens might turn to reckless behavior and others might withdraw or blithely insist that "everything's fine." There is no right or wrong way to grieve.

There will also be different responses to a loss in the same household, Edelman told me, because "if the child just lost a grandparent, that means one of the parents just lost a parent." This is a good time to enlist trusted friends, teachers, coaches, neighbors, or extended family to be extra support in your kids' lives. Edelman shared that when kids experience loss, they need at least one adult who gives them "permission and space to talk about their feelings," but that person doesn't have to be a parent, at least not right away. A loving community can help kids know that all of their emotions and reactions are normal. When Edelman's kids were young, she would talk it through with them in simple ways: "When something sad happens, it's okay to be sad. When I'm sad, I cry. It's okay for you to do that too."

Also, grief isn't time-limited, so if your kids find themselves sad at unexpected moments, Edelman says it can help to share the message that "it doesn't mean that you got grief wrong—it means that you really loved that person and you really miss them."

Post-Traumatic Growth

One of awe's healing powers is this: Awe allows us to experience beauty and joy without denying more challenging emotions like grief and loneliness. On the anniversary of a loss, we can *also* notice the sunrise or appreciate the friend who remembered and checked in with us.

A few months after my dad died, I rushed out the door to get to school before my students. It was a bitingly cold December morning, and my heart felt raw with grief. And then I saw it: a single rosebud on a scraggly bush in front of our house. I began to laugh and then cry at the absurdity of such a lovely little thing proclaiming its place in the dark world. No, this little bud did not make things all better. It wasn't a cure for sadness. But it reminded me that my heart was capable of feeling more than grief; there was also room for surprise and delight. It reminded me that I am big enough to house multiple emotions at once.

Edelman, who has spent years researching the aftereffects of childhood loss, offers these words of hope for parents worried about their children: "I want parents to know that a child can experience a loss—even a major one—when they're young and still have a beautiful, rich, and fulfilling life as an adult. It will be something they carry with them forever. They will carry that memory forward, but that memory will often enrich their lives in ways that you can't even imagine now."

Her reflection is rooted in a concept called *post-traumatic growth*. Psychologists Richard Tedeschi and Lawrence Calhoun coined this term in the 1990s to describe how people can experience positive growth after enduring a psychological struggle. As Tedeschi told the American Psychological Association's *Monitor on Psychology*, people often "develop new understandings of themselves, the world they live in, how to relate to other people, the kind of future they might have, and a better understanding of how to live life."[9]

In Edelman's research, she spoke with hundreds of adults who lost a parent during childhood and found that many, over time, came to see their traumatic experience as a "springboard to a form of personal growth, and that includes, oftentimes, an enhanced sense of meaning or purpose in your own life." They came to a place where they could say things like, "I was able to grow from my experience in *this* way." "I became resilient, and it helped me deal with this other challenge in my life." "This loss helped me put things in perspective. I began to understand what's important and what's not; what's worth getting upset about and what's not."

When I share this research with teens, I add that this doesn't mean we are supposed to feel grateful for the hardships themselves. We don't need to jump to silver linings while swallowing our pain. Rather, it means that in the aftermath of life's inevitable challenges, we can find ways to integrate our losses into the fabric of our life stories. Humans have an awe-inspiring capacity to make meaning out of struggle.

Bittersweet Wonder: A Conversation with Susan Cain

When I read Susan Cain's Bittersweet: How Sorrow and Longing Make Us Whole, *I felt awe repeatedly: tears, chills, and whoas that made me feel deeply connected to our collective humanity. I had to pause multiple times to sit and savor her words and what they might mean for my parenting.*

I had the opportunity to interview Cain for KQED's MindShift, and so I asked her how her research might apply to those raising kids. I'm grateful to MindShift for letting me share this interview in full.

Kris: In the first section of your book, you describe some of the "uses of sadness," from sharpening our attention to stimulating creativity. I really love this line: "If we could honor sadness a little more, maybe we could see it—rather than enforced smiles or righteous outrage—as the bridge we need to connect with one another." What do you mean by that, and what's its application to raising kids?

Cain: None of us wants to see our kids sad, of course. At the same time, it is a deeply human experience. So telegraphing to our kids that they shouldn't feel sad is not only not helpful, but it makes them feel shame on top of whatever they're feeling sad about.

But in terms of honoring sadness as a bridge, we are deeply evolutionarily primed to respond to each other's sadness. When you see another being in trouble or crying, your vagus nerve reacts to that. This instinct to feel bad when we see somebody else feeling bad—and to want to do something about it—is as much a part of humanity as our need to breathe.

Kris: For teens, the pressure to bounce back quickly and show that something didn't really affect them can be intense. You write about the distinction between "moving on" and "moving forward." Can you talk about that?

Cain: The phrases *Move on* and *Get over it* are basically saying, "It's not okay for you to carry your loss for very long. Sure, it's okay to be sad on the day of the loss. And maybe it's okay the day after that. But there's a point at which we are going to expect you to get over it. It should no longer be part of you. Go back to your pre-loss self."

But there's another path: You can move forward with your life and carry that loss with you. You can still feel sad sometimes while also integrating new experiences and having new joys. It all becomes part of you. So instead of saying, "Okay, I've got to get from sad back to happy as fast as I can," you realize life is just a collection of experiences that shape you and you're carrying them all.

Kris: While reading your book, I wrote in the margins this phrase from Susan David: "Life's beauty is inseparable from its fragility." As adults, we sometimes struggle with how to talk to kids about the fragile side of life—and put a premium on shielding them from pain and discomfort. What are some of your thoughts about this?

Cain: I think we inadvertently teach kids, especially those growing up in relative comfort, that "normal" means everything is sky high and flourishing. But the smooth road is not the default; it's the detour. Unexpected twists and turns are actually the main road. When life seems to go off path, kids need to know that it doesn't mean something is wrong with them or with their experiences. It's incredibly comforting for children to know that life is made up of bittersweet. The question then becomes, how do you navigate it? Challenges can become an opportunity for them to learn—while still under the loving guidance of their parents—that this is part of what life is.

When my kids were little, we rented a house in the countryside that was right next to a field where two donkeys lived—Lucky and Norman. The kids and the donkeys absolutely fell in love with each other. They spent their whole week feeding the donkeys apples and carrots. And then, as always happens with any summer romance, it had to come to an end. The kids were crying themselves to sleep at the thought of having to say goodbye to Lucky and Norman. We said all kinds of things to help them feel better. But what gave them the most comfort was when we said, "These kinds of goodbyes are a natural part of life. It's not the first time you're saying them, and it's not going to be the last time. Everybody has to say these kinds of goodbyes. It's natural." It helped them to hear that the feelings they were having were normal.

Kris: Just last night, my eight-year-old son called me into his room in tears at 10 p.m. and said, "I don't want to fall asleep because once I do, vacation's over." It strikes me that these small transitions can be a fertile time for parents and teachers to help kids think about the beauty in the bittersweet.

Cain: Absolutely. Because transitions are mini goodbyes, right? They're an expression of the final goodbye that we all face eventually. We don't know that when we're getting upset about the transition, but that's really what's happening. And so every time you can walk your child through the discomfort of transitions and the pain of the mini goodbye—whether it's the last day of camp or the last day of vacation—those are prime learning moments.

I quote a poem in the book by Gerard Manley Hopkin called "Spring and Fall." And it's written by the poet to a little girl who is crying because the leaves are falling and she doesn't want the leaves to go away. She doesn't want winter to come. And he says, "Márgarét, áre you gríeving / Over Goldengrove unleaving?" And then later he says, "It ís the blight that man was born for, / It is Margaret you mourn for."

I can't say those lines without shivers because of the wisdom and the empathy of that insight: Margaret doesn't know it yet; she's crying over the fact that life is impermanent.

But here's the thing that's also true about that impermanence: It can be so painful, but it's also so intensely beautiful. The beauty of impermanence might be the greatest beauty we have—and all humans experience it. There's something about knowing that we're all in this crazy, beautiful, intensely imperfect experience together that is very uplifting.

A Final Thought

I often talk to my kids about my paternal grandmother, their great-grandmother. Grandma died a week before I left for college, and when I describe her to people, I sometimes say, "She never met a creature she couldn't talk to—human, cat, dog, or bird." Let me tell you a bit of her story.

On February 1, 1919, Eliza Ellen turned four years old. Twenty days later, she lost her mom. The third wave of the influenza pandemic had found its way to the backwoods of Monroe County, Arkansas. Her mother, Marie, was thirty-nine when she died, leaving behind six children. Eliza and her siblings still had their father, but he was emotionally and financially ill-equipped to care for the children. He began to leave them alone for days and then weeks at a stretch. Grandma remembered subsisting on stale crackers and currant jelly. Eventually, the state stepped in, and the children were sent to live in St. Joseph's Orphanage in Little Rock. Her siblings were quickly adopted. Eliza was not.

When Eliza turned eighteen, she boarded a bus and made her way to California, where she found a job as a waitress. One day, my grandfather walked into her diner and ordered a cup of coffee from her. Three weeks later, they got married.

I loved visiting my grandparents when I was a kid. Their run-down, two-bedroom Los Angeles home sheltered a dozen cats, a few birds, and a lumbering basset hound. Every morning, Grandma would get up early to walk around the block, feeding stray animals and checking in on her neighbors. She was everyone's grandma. Birds came when she whistled, and squirrels ate out of her hand. She never received a formal education, but she sent her son to college. She didn't drive, but she once took a dozen buses around Los Angeles hunting for the sold-out Cabbage Patch doll I wanted for my eighth birthday. Shortly before she died, she made my dad promise he'd find homes for all twelve of her cats. He did.

History doesn't have discrete start and end dates. Events ripple forward. What was set in motion in February 1919 laps at my ankles over one hundred years later. That four-year-old girl survived the loss of her mom. And then survived again and again and again, enduring challenges I hope my children never face—and yet possessing a resilience, compassion, and fierce joy I want to pass on to them.

My social media feed is filled with parenting advice. But when I turn inward to listen, I can almost hear Grandma whispering: *Slow down. These years don't last as long as you think they will. Just look at those beautiful faces. It's okay if they are extra needy today. It's okay if you are cranky. If they feel loved at the end of the day, you've done enough.*

5 Wonderful Ways to Help Kids Understand the Lifespan

1. Tell Kids Their Origin Story. Share with your kids the story of how they came to you—their birth or adoption. Look through baby pictures and tell them stories about all those wonderful firsts: first smile, first word, first song that made them kick their feet, first time tasting a lemon, first day of school. Let them hear your wonder about who they have been at every age and stage.

2. Look Through Family Photos. "Want to see what Grandma looked like when she was your age?" "Have you seen the picture of Uncle Ramon's high school garage band?" "Here's the enlistment picture of your great-grandpa who you never got to meet." "Look at you! Can you believe you were ever that little?" Family photos build connections and offer clear examples of the arc of life.

3. Foster Multigenerational Memories. Kids and older adults have a lot to offer one another. Are there older adults in your extended family who could serve as mentors to your kids—in person or through video calls? Is there a senior center in town where your teen could offer tech support and build connections? Is there an older neighbor who could use a dinner invitation? Get creative in finding ways to bring generations together.

4. Interview Living History. Is your kid studying space in school? Encourage them to ask Grandpa about the moon landing. Does your kid love piano? Put them in touch with that retired concert pianist who lives in town. One day when my kids were asking me about farm life, I suddenly remembered that we had an expert in the family: Grandma grew up on a ranch! Through FaceTime, Grandma gamely fielded a dozen questions about milking cows, gathering eggs, making butter, and riding horses.

5. Seek Out New Life. There's nothing like holding a baby or stroking a puppy to evoke the "aww!" in awe. Visit a local farm in the spring to see baby goats, chicks, and sheep. Keep an eye on the nest some swallows built on your balcony. Ask a friend if your kids can come visit their new puppy. Give your teens any opportunity to interact with little kids—to experience children looking up at them with wide eyes and testing them with exuberant energy.

10 Awe-Inspiring Picture Books About Life and Loss

Fletcher and the Falling Leaves **by Julia Rawlinson and Tiphanie Beeke.** Fletcher the fox is experiencing his first autumn. When leaves begin to fall from his favorite tree, he becomes very worried. But he learns that there is unexpected beauty in each season.

In Every Life **by Marla Frazee.** This simple, luscious book reads like a poem, or a prayer. It starts with celebrating birth and then captures the wondrous moments "in every life."

Memories of a Birch Tree **by Daniel Cañas and Blanca Millán.** A birch tree is uprooted from the forest and planted in a city. Told from the perspective of the tree, the book shows how he adjusts to his new life and finds unexpected ways to give and receive.

Remembering Sundays with Grandpa **by Lauren H. Kerstein and Nanette Regan.** Written by a child psychologist, this book follows Henry and his mom as they navigate their grief over the loss of Grandpa. They take solace in concrete memories—like the stories he read aloud in his rocking chair and the jewelry box he used to wind up so they could dance.

Still This Love Goes On **by Buffy Sainte-Marie and Julie Flett.** This book is based on Buffy Sainte-Marie's award-winning song of the same name. Both the author and illustrator are Cree, and the words and pictures offer an Indigenous perspective on nature, seasons, love, and loss.

You'll Find Me **by Amanda Rawson Hill and Joanne Lew-Vriethoff.** This book approaches the death of a loved one with tenderness and simplicity, with an omnipresent narrator using a refrain, "I will not always be . . . But you'll find me . . ." to show both what is lost and what lives on when someone dies.

The Heart and the Bottle **by Oliver Jeffers.** This gorgeous book tells the story of a little girl who delights in exploring the world with her grandfather. But suddenly, his chair is empty, so she puts her heart in a bottle and loses her sense of wonder until a new friend helps her free her heart.

The Invisible String **by Patrice Karst and Joanne Lew-Vriethoff.** This classic book celebrates all the ways we are tied to those we love. "An Invisible String made of love. Even though you can't see it with your eyes, you can feel it deep in your heart, and know that you are always connected to the ones you love."

I Love You All the Time **by Deborah Farmer Kris and Jennifer Zivoin.** This book is based on my nighttime refrain to my children when they were young: "I love you when you're happy. I love you when you're sad. I love you when you're feeling scared. I love you when you're mad. I love you all the time."

Hundred: What You Learn in a Lifetime **by Heike Faller and Valerio Vidali.** A two-hundred-page picture book? Yes, because each two-page spread covers one year of life—and one thing a person might learn at age three, thirty-three, or ninety-three. A stunning look at a lifetime of learning!

CHAPTER SEVEN

THE WONDER OF HUMAN KINDNESS

My wish for you is that you continue. Continue to be who and how you are, to astonish a mean world with your acts of kindness.

—Maya Angelou

Seventh grade started on a rough note for me. I moved from the comfort of a neighborhood school to the city's junior high, which housed over a thousand students. I felt lost and scared much of the time.

Sometimes I would hop off the bus in the afternoon, jump on my bike, and pedal down to the elementary school. "Do you need any help?" I would ask my former sixth grade teacher. Ms. Park would smile and say, "I would love some."

I would then spend an hour washing chalkboards, correcting spelling tests, or pumping up rubber kickballs. I don't remember if we talked much about my feelings or worries, but Ms. Park seemed to sense why I was there. Susan David, author of *Emotional Agility*, once told me, "When children and adolescents are very upset, literally just the presence of a loving person helps to deescalate and creates the space where calm is invited in." Ms. Park was that loving person.

That's why, in college, I sent Ms. Park a card on Mother's Day one year to thank her for her kindness during that pivotal time. She was one of the reasons I wanted to become a teacher: I wanted to be that type of presence for kids. I don't know if Ms. Park's kindness at the time made me feel awe, but the *memories* of it certainly have—over and over—in the years that followed.

Ms. Park isn't the only recipient of a much-delayed thank-you letter. I've long been interested in the research on gratitude. According to a Harvard Medical School research summary, gratitude is an emotion that helps people "feel more positive emotions, relish good experiences, improve their health, deal with adversity, and build strong relationships."[1] One study asked participants to write a thank-you letter to someone who had made a difference—explaining why they were thankful in *concrete* terms. Just writing the letter is powerful, but *delivering* the letter led to improved emotional health six months later.[2] In a follow-up study of adolescents, the teens who experienced the greatest emotional benefit from delivering gratitude letters were the ones who initially had the lowest levels of "positive affect." As the researchers wrote, "It makes sense that youth with little exposure to positive emotions might be the most inspired and changed by the experience. This might be due to an epiphany, a sudden feeling of insight."[3] In other words, it might be due to feeling awe.

A few years ago, I shared this study with some teens, and I invited them to write and deliver their own thank-you letters. As a model, I wrote to two other people who made a difference during those awkward first months of middle school.

> Dear Alison and Emily,
>
> I've been talking about gratitude with some students this week, and my mind keeps wandering back to the two of you. I guess that's a sign that I need to say a proper thank-you for changing my life two-plus decades ago.
>
> My very first week at junior high was objectively terrible. Because of a travel issue, I missed the first day of school. When I arrived on day two, I couldn't open my locker. I was yelled at for being late to homeroom and then struggled for the

rest of the day to find both my classes and a friendly face. I was more successful with the former than the latter. To make matters worse, when I got my back-to-school haircut, I'd said *bob*, but the hairdresser heard *buzz*. Okay, it was more like a pixie-cut, but it was not what I had wanted, and it added to the screaming mess of awkwardness that was ME.

And then there was Mrs. T's English class, where a couple boys sat behind me, throwing wads of paper at my head and whispering, "Is it a boy or a girl?" day after day after day. At some point, I just tried to make myself invisible.

But one day, the two of you waved me over to your desks. You told me to ignore those kids. You said, "Ask Mrs. T. if she will move your seat near us." And when I hesitated—because, honestly, my confidence was pretty shaky at that point—you went up yourselves and asked for me.

My memories of you both after that moment are consistently awesome, but all those good memories began in that moment when you reached outside your circle and drew me in, when you gave me an escape hatch from a frankly scary situation, when you let me borrow your courage and helped me re-find my voice.

I have spent most of the last two decades teaching in middle and high schools. And when I see a student reach out and draw someone else in, I think of you every single time. Thank you for being those people in that moment. I am forever grateful.

When Emily wrote back to me, she confessed that she didn't remember asking the teacher to switch my desk, just the friendship that followed. She then added, "I read your letter to my kids—to remind them that they never know how their actions will touch other people."

And the Number-One Source of Awe Is . . .

According to the data, the most common source of awe is noticing the goodness of other people. "It's kindness and courage," Dacher Keltner told me. "We really have this capacity to be moved by other people." As he wrote in an article for *Greater Good Magazine*:[4]

> What most commonly led people to feel awe? Nature? Spiritual practice? Listening to music? In fact, it was other people's courage, kindness, strength, or overcoming—actions of strangers, roommates, teachers, colleagues at work, people in the news, characters on podcasts, and our neighbors and family members. Around the world, we are most likely to feel awe when moved by moral beauty: exceptional virtue, character, and ability, marked by a purity and goodness of intention and action.
>
> Over 95 percent of the moral beauty that stirred awe worldwide was in actions people took on behalf of others.

In an era marked by division, I find it profoundly hopeful that we are drawn to human goodness. Seeing other people act in brave and compassionate ways evokes wonder. It gives us goosebumps. It moves us to tears. Even the memory of a past kindness—like two classmates getting the seating chart changed—can offer a spark of warmth during cold seasons of life. We've all told our children some version of the sentiment that *a little kindness goes a long way*. Maybe they need us to go a step further and back it up with stories from our own lives about small kindnesses that made a big difference.

A Few Things We Know About Kids, Kindness, and Awe

Feeling awe prompts people to be kind and generous. You'll recall from chapter 1 that staring at tall trees made people more likely to help a stranger who dropped their belongings than staring at a building. Writing about a moment of awe made people more willing to volunteer than writing about a moment of happiness.

Does this translate to kids? Researchers in the Netherlands asked that same question. In two studies of eight- to thirteen-year-old children, researchers examined whether awe could promote children's kindness toward refugee families.[5] The kids were divided into three groups to watch one of three video clips—an awe-inspiring scene, a joy-inspiring scene, and a neutral, mundane scene.

As researchers wrote, "Results showed that experiences of awe more than joy led children to spend their time counting food items for refugee families as well as to donate items they had earned (a raffle ticket and a chocolate snack) to refugee children. Moreover, children who watched the awe-eliciting clip showed greater parasympathetic nervous system activation, which is known to facilitate calm social engagement. Awe, an aesthetic and moral emotion, helps societies flourish by making children more generous." The report continues, "Although children from an early age are more likely to help in-group than out-group members, our findings show that awe can open them up to helping members of a national minority."

Other research points to the role kindness plays in bolstering our physical health. According to Stanford's James Doty, modern humans often live in "threat mode." We are overstimulated and on constant alert because of pressures and stressors. When our nervous system is in this mode, it taxes our immune system. Acting with compassion, Doty says, can reset our body's systems. He writes, "When someone acts with compassionate intentions, this has a huge, huge positive effect on their physiology. It takes them out of threat mode and puts them into the rest and digest mode."[6]

Being kind also supports our mental health. A 2022 study out of Ohio State University found that performing acts of kindness eased the symptoms of people struggling with moderate to severe anxiety or depression.[7] Participants were split into three groups. One group was tasked with planning and taking part in two weekly social activities. The second group practiced cognitive reappraisal (e.g., identifying and revising negative thought patterns). The third group was told to perform three acts of kindness daily for two days out of the week. This kindness group reported doing things such as baking cookies for friends and leaving encouraging sticky notes for a roommate.

Every single one of these techniques helped reduce depressive symptoms. But only "acts of kindness" *also* increased people's sense of social connection. And that's important! According to study coauthor David Cregg, "Social connection is one of the ingredients of life most strongly associated with well-being. Performing acts of kindness seems to be one of the best ways to promote those connections."[8]

Cregg's coauthor, Jennifer Cheavens, told *Ohio State News*, "We often think that people with depression have enough to deal with, so we don't want to burden them by asking them to help others. But these results run counter to that," she said. "Doing nice things for people and focusing on the needs of others may actually help people with depression and anxiety feel better about themselves."[9]

When I spoke to Harvard "happiness researcher" Robert Waldinger, he echoed the importance of social connection. According to Waldinger's research, "the people who were most satisfied in their relationships at age fifty were the healthiest (mentally and physically) at age eighty." Relationships require tending, Waldinger told me, and people who have the strongest relationships are "proactive, reaching out rather than just assuming that friendships are going to take care of themselves." Helping kids build relationship skills early can put them on a path of flourishing.

How can parents help set kids down this path? We can help them "find the helpers," and we can help them *become* the helpers.

Finding the Helpers

Fred Rogers famously described how noticing goodness can be emotionally protective for children when they encounter the darker side of humanity. In an interview, he said, "My mother used to say . . . whenever there would be any real catastrophe that was in the movies or on the air, she would say: 'Always look for the helpers. There will always be helpers.'"[10]

Versions of Rogers's quote are often shared when tragic events hit the headlines. But what if we shared these helper stories with our kids more regularly? What if we told them about the stranger who helped us jumpstart our car or carry our groceries? What if we mentioned the coworker who offered to make copies for us when we were running late? Or the neighbor who brought out our trash bins when we forgot? What if, in our families, communicating these "kindness moments," and the awe they inspire, became the norm?

Kindness rarely makes the news, so we must actively bring human goodness to the attention of our kids. They are bombarded with lopsided data about the state of the world: a steady diet of headlines about school shootings, political division, violent crime, greed, poverty, and climate disasters. Fred Rogers wrote, "The media shows the tiniest percentage of what people do. There are millions and millions of people doing wonderful things all over the world, and they're generally not the ones being touted in the news."[11]

I am not suggesting that we keep our kids uninformed about the world. An educated citizenry is vital to society. Instead, I'm advocating giving them a fulsome vision of this world—including how people's courage, integrity, compassion, and perseverance help shape it.

We know that kids and teens are anxious about the state of the world. In one survey of young adults, nearly 60 percent said that they felt "very or extremely worried" about climate change.[12] A study out of the Harvard Kennedy School reported that 40 percent of young adults (eighteen- to thirty-year-olds) were concerned about becoming victims of gun violence, and 47 percent of this same group reported "feeling down, depressed, or hopeless."[13] Feelings of helplessness and hopelessness can be paralyzing, and they are at odds with thriving.

Jamil Zaki is the director of the Stanford Social Neuroscience Lab and author of the book *Hope for Cynics: The Surprising Science of Human Goodness*. He told me that sometimes adults "try to keep our kids safe by making them feel unsafe"—warning them of dangers and threats. But this can have unintended consequences for children's mental and emotional well-being, Zaki said. "If we focus kids on the negative— on the worst parts of life and the worst parts of humanity—we're going to end up shrinking their world, making it harder for them to trust, and making it harder for them to explore, take risks, and form relationships."

Here is something else Zaki told me: Humans tend to *underestimate* human goodness. Take this study as an example: A group of researchers "dropped" nearly 17,000 wallets in forty countries over the course of two years. Some wallets had no money, some had the equivalent of $13, and some had the equivalent of $100. The wallets all contained contact information for the "owner." So how many people attempted to reach the owner of the lost wallet? Researchers assumed that the higher the amount of money in the wallet, the less likely the wallet was to be returned. And a poll of 279 "top-performing academic economists" agreed. Humans are greedy, right? But the exact opposite turned out to be true. Forty-six percent of empty wallets were reported, compared with 61 percent of $13 wallets and 72 percent of $100 wallets. The more money that was lost, the more often people went out of their way to return the money to the owner. People *wanted* to help out strangers they had never met.[14]

Zaki was not surprised by this, because his research has found that "most people value compassion over selfishness." This is important information. If our kids believe that the majority of people simply don't care about pressing issues, it's easy to feel hopeless. And yet "there are many ways that our kids are probably part of a supermajority that they don't know they're part of," said Zaki. "If you know that most people want, just like you do, a more peaceful, egalitarian, and sustainable world, then fighting for it makes a lot more sense."

I think novelist John Green was onto something when he said this on an episode of the *Freakonomics* podcast: "A lot of times good news happens slowly and bad news happens all at once. And so we tend to focus on the bad news that's crashing over us in waves, and not on the slow, long-term work that people are doing together to try to make a better world for us to share."[15]

Turning Toward Goodness

When my kids were little, we had a Thankful Jar on the kitchen table. Here's how I described our nightly ritual in a PBS KIDS column:[16]

> The materials are bare bones: a jar and a bag of glass beads I picked up at a craft store. Each night, we take turns sharing something that we are thankful for, asking ourselves, *What made me smile today? What went well? Who helped me?* The kids took to it instantly. Each night at dinnertime, the five-year-old enthusiastically brings the jar and bag to the table and announces who gets to go first.
>
> The two-year-old is often grateful for the items he sees on his dinner plate: "I thankful for avocado and chicken nuggets and apples." His older sister's expressions have become increasingly complex over time. She talks about people who helped her at school, an activity she enjoyed, and simple moments of pleasure such as dancing with her brother or picking flowers. It's been a wonderful window into what brings her joy—particularly as she regularly expresses gratitude for snuggling with her family. As for the parents? Well, on days when work has been stressful or

car repairs have been costly, this simple exercise has been good for us, too, as we pause to remind ourselves of the goodness that fills our lives.

After three or four years, we stopped using this jar regularly. Old rituals pave the way for new ones. But when my now-middle-school daughter found the jar in the back of a cabinet, she wouldn't let me discard it. The memories attached to it were just too wonderful.

In her book *How to Be a Happier Parent*, KJ Dell'Antonia offers this insight: "Humans are hardwired to focus on the negative. When we train our brains to notice and absorb everyday pleasures—the moments when we are safe and snug and warm with our families around us—we gain a deeper reservoir of joy to bolster us when things get rough."[17] Zaki describes this as "social savoring"—or "noticing the good stuff as it happens." He said that savoring small moments of human goodness helps us correct the negativity bias that most of us are prone to. "I try do this with my kids all the time," said Zaki. "I share with them if I notice somebody doing something really kind, and I ask them [to] tell me about the kind thing that somebody in [their] class did." Social savoring, over time, "becomes a habit of mind."

That's why most nights, after the kids are in bed but before they are asleep, I hang out for a moment and tell them something from the day that I noticed about them—a small "something good." It can be as simple as, *Thanks again for walking the dog this morning before school. I know it was cold outside.* Or, *Hey, I know your sibling was bothering you tonight— and you kept it in check. I appreciate it.* Beyond ensuring that my kids know I see the best in them, these evening check-ins have also helped my parenting. I'm primed to look for my kids' moments of goodness because I want to share them. When we intentionally look for goodness in others, we are more likely to see it.

According to relationship researcher John Gottman, the "magic ratio" of positive to negative feedback is 5:1—five positive interactions to every negative interaction.[18] Kids often feel like adults only notice when they "mess up," not when they try, so they grow wary of feedback. If you know you need to correct your kid, it helps to be mindful about also giving them positive feedback. These positive interactions say to kids, *I see you. Not only that, I see the best in you.*

In Praise of "Tiny Kindness"

In 2019, illness invaded our house and shredded my make-the-holidays-magical to-do list. No decorating sugar cookies or wrapping homemade caramels in wax paper squares. No caroling or visiting lights displays.

And yet.

On Christmas Eve, a friend left a pot of spaghetti on the doorstep for our dinner. A former student brought over a five-hundred-piece puzzle to keep the kids occupied while I wrestled with health insurance calls and caught up on laundry. A sibling dropped everything and traveled two hundred miles to help us out. I can't think about that year without grateful tears coming to my eyes.

A few years later, something similar happened. Sickness struck, canceling highly anticipated plans. But once again, helpers came through. Like the local shop owner who wrapped the gifts I'd ordered and dropped them off on my doorstep on Christmas Eve—along with a bag of cough drops and a tin of homemade treats. Just like moments of goodness in our kids, acts of compassion are so easy to find once we start looking for them. Remember, awe can be an everyday emotion, not a once-in-a-blue-moon feeling. Dramatic stories of human virtue are wonderful. But what if we also looked for tiny kindnesses?

A few years ago, my friend Rachel Hunt started a social media project called Tiny Kindness. As she shared: "I started it in my grief, on the approximate one-year anniversary of my brother's burial. I suddenly had a desperate need to consciously look for goodness and kindness in the world. So I put out a call on social media and asked friends to send short stories of small acts of kindness they've received that felt big to them. And they did."[19]

I sent in one of the first Tiny Kindness stories describing an act of kindness from my second year of teaching. The memory still gives me goosebumps. The post read:

> Once, when life was overwhelming, I kept putting off dinner invitations from a good friend. I just didn't have the emotional energy for social stuff outside of work. One day, she quietly left a package at my front door. Five labeled paper bags: Deborah's Lunch Monday, Deborah's Lunch Tuesday, Deborah's Lunch Wednesday . . . Every day that week, I ate a healthy lunch (a rarity) and cried in gratitude.

I love that Rachel's work highlights the "types of kindness that feel small to the person giving them, but not at all small to the person receiving them." She continues: "It's kindness that takes place after infertility, miscarriages, births, illness, divorce, and death; on doorsteps, buses, subways, airplanes, and at grocery stores; between strangers, neighbors, friends, and family members. It is instance after instance of humans showing up for each other in beautiful ways. These kindnesses are happening everywhere, all of the time."[20]

Like this story someone submitted, which encapsulates so much of what I love about New York City:

> My five-year-old son polished off a banana on the subway and handed me the peel to hold for the rest of our long trip uptown. A young man getting off at the next stop noticed, took the peel from me, and dropped it in the trash on his way off the platform.

A couple of years ago, I shared several Tiny Kindness posts with a class of seventh graders and invited them to write one of their own—to describe a moment when someone offered them kindness that made a difference.

I adore middle schoolers, but I also know this is an age when they are pulling away from their parents and toward their peers. So I was surprised that most of their stories were about their parents. Like these two:

> My mom noticed I was having a bad day, so she made me a cup of tea and put it on my bedside table.

> When I messed up on my science poster, my dad stayed up late helping me cut out and glue stuff on a new one.

Parents of adolescents: This is your much-needed reminder that your kids crave the kindness you offer them, even when they don't seem to care.

Helping our kids notice the goodness of others is one way to access the protective benefits of awe. But it's not enough to just help them see the helpers; we can also teach them to *be* the helpers.

"Once I was at the deli ordering my breakfast when a lady came up to me and paid for everything I got. She told me that she paid for my items because she wanted to remind me that whenever I feel alone, I can remember that someone will always be there for me, and that God will never leave my side. She also reminded me that even though I may see other people doing the wrong thing, I should always remember to keep my priorities straight and my future as my main focus."—Riley, middle schooler

Becoming the Helpers

Awe pulls us out of ourselves—and this stepping *back* from the self can help our kids step *toward* others. Let me tell you about one such full-circle moment.

When my son was in third grade, he played on a multiage basketball team of mostly eight- to ten-year-olds. When they entered their first game of the season, they encountered a team stacked with middle schoolers.

The score was lopsided from the beginning—partly because the other team had a seventh grader who downed three-pointers like Stephen Curry. But then something extraordinary happened. A kid on my son's team missed a shot. The opposing seventh-grade wunderkind grabbed the rebound, but he did not send it down the court. Instead, he handed it back to the young shooter—a kid still learning how to dribble—and encouraged him to take another shot. Everyone else had already run downcourt, leaving just these two players beneath the basket. We all watched as the kid threw up the ball again. Swish. His mouth dropped open in astonishment. The seventh-grade opponent high-fived him, and the parents and players on both sides stood and cheered.

On the way home, my son didn't talk about the final score (his team lost by double digits). He only wanted to talk about that moment: "Did you see what that tall kid did? He was such a good player, but he let Kace take that shot! That was so nice of him! I mean, that was the best part of the whole game!"

A few months later, my son was playing a flag football game against a different school. Again, both teams were multiage, but this time my son's team had the overall age advantage. In the game's last minutes, my son's coach pulled the team together for a quiet conversation. Would they consider letting a younger, smaller player on the other team score a touchdown—even though that meant they might lose the game? They agreed, and I'll never forget the look of wonder on that child's face as he ran into the end zone.

Why did my son's team do this? In part, it was because they remembered what that basketball player had done for their teammate and how good it felt. As Fred Rogers reminds us, "All of us, at some time or other, need help. Whether we're giving or receiving help, each one of us has something valuable to bring to this world. That's one of the things that connects us as neighbors—in our own way, each one of us is a giver and a receiver."[21]

Kids' brains are hardwired for empathy. Research suggests that most humans have an innate capacity to step into another person's shoes and respond to their emotions.[22] As Susan Cain notes in *Bittersweet*, "Our nervous systems make little distinction between our own pain and the pain of others, it turns out; they react similarly to both. This instinct is as much a part of us as the desire to eat and breathe. The compassionate instinct is also a fundamental aspect of the human success story."[23]

This insight reminded me of a conversation with Richard Weissbourd,[24] director of Harvard's Making Caring Common project. He told me, "Almost all kids are kind to *somebody* and have empathy for *somebody*. The real work is getting them to be kind and empathetic to people outside of their immediate circle of concern."

Kids of all ages, and especially young children, may need support with "putting other people on their radar," Weissbourd told me. It takes practice to get in the habit of noticing the needs of people outside our inner circle. As a starting place for helping your child grow this empathy, you can point out the kid on the playground who may not be playing with any of the other kids or ask your child to tell you about a new classmate—and then talk about how to welcome them.

Kids and adults alike are "more distressed when we feel helpless and passive—and more comfortable when we are taking action," said Weissbourd. Because of their natural empathetic impulses, kids may feel upset when they see a classmate being picked on or hear about people who are struggling. Adults can help them "turn passivity into activity."

For example, young children may not know what to do if someone gets hurt at the park, but if adults encourage them to "tell a parent or tell a teacher," then children will develop the habit of acting when they see someone in need. Likewise, when children help you choose food and clothing to donate to a community agency—or when they come with you to check on an elderly or sick neighbor—they begin to tune in to the needs of others. As Weissbourd said, regular moments of family service "create an expectation that this is what we do."

As kids get older and are seeking more independence from us and time with friends, we can encourage them to join in on group service initiatives where they get to work with peers toward a common goal: organizing a drive, participating in a run or walk for a cause, cleaning up a public park, or tutoring younger students. A 2023 study in the *Journal of the American Medical Association* analyzed survey data from parents of over 50,000 kids and teens across the United States. They found that "volunteering was associated with higher odds of excellent or very good health and flourishing in children and adolescents, and with lower odds of anxiety in adolescents and behavioral problems in children and adolescents" as reported by their parents.[25]

How Parents Can Confront the Crisis of Kindness

According to science journalist and parenting writer Melinda Wenner Moyer, the United States is facing a "crisis of kindness." Moyer went searching for ways to help our kids counteract the forces that drag us down and wrote about her findings in the book *How to Raise Kids Who Aren't A**holes: Science-Based Strategies for Better Parenting—from Tots to Teens.*

Moyer found this: If we want to raise kind kids, we have to attend to their emotional development. As she told me, "Over and over again, I saw studies that pointed out that just talking about feelings—allowing kids to have their feelings—is an important foundation for the development of generosity."

Kids may be hardwired for empathy, but it is still a skill they need to develop. And adults play a key role in nurturing this skill. Emotional self-awareness is a building block for empathy, as is talking with kids about the link between their actions and another person's reactions. "In order to be kind and helpful to someone else, you have to first be able to perceive what another person is feeling—and how what you do can directly affect another person's state of mind," said Moyer. "Help kids understand that there is a direct connection between what we do and what other people feel."

This practical empathy can help kids avoid hurting others, and it can also help them reach out proactively. For children, that might look like this: *My classmate seems sad. What can I do to help them not feel as sad?* When parents regularly talk with kids about what kindness looks like and how their actions affect other people, they raise kids who are less likely to bully and more likely to stand up for others.

Moyer pointed to this study as an example: Fourth and fifth graders whose parents gave them clear advice about what to do when they saw bullying were much more likely to reach out and support bullying victims.[26] "Kids do actually listen to their parents," said Moyer. "Having these conversations changes how our kids behave and the choices they make at school."

So what should kids do if they see another child being picked on? We can teach them to reach out to that child—sit with them at lunch, invite them to play at recess, or even just stand near them warmly. In surveys, children who have been bullied report that "the most helpful thing that other kids did after they've been bullied was to listen to them and to spend time with them," said Moyer. "If your child feels courageous enough to say something to [the child who is bullying], that's great. But if they don't, there's still so much they can do to be supportive."

Moyer also reminds parents that kids are incredible observers of adult behavior. When you make a mistake or say something unkind—as we all do at times—that can be a teachable moment. "When I lose my temper, I will use that as a conversation starter later and say, *Gosh. I got really angry there. And I think I should've taken some deep breaths before I said what I said*," she explained. "And sometimes I ask my kids, *What do you think I could have done better in that situation?* It's all about modeling what you want to see while also showing that you're still growing and learning from your mistakes. We're all human, and that's okay."

Toddsgiving: Laura's Story

As I was drafting this chapter, I got a message from my friend Laura Zaks, reminding me to perform an act of kindness on November 19 in honor of her brother, who died from cancer as a teenager on that date. Laura's family calls it Toddsgiving, and she explains the ritual like this:

Toddsgiving is a way to put some purpose behind my tears. Prior to starting the November 19 tradition, I would find myself wanting to isolate on that day. I didn't feel right going about a regular routine when the day felt anything but regular. It was just too much.

When I had my own kids, that feeling changed. I knew that I wanted them to know the uncle they'd never meet, and I knew that the only way I could do that was to make them a part of what Todd did best: making people smile.

Toddsgiving was born out of my desire to show my kids that even on our worst days, we can make someone else feel good. We started small. That first year, I let my oldest child decide what we should do. As a New England donut-loving kid, he suggested we drive through every Dunkin' Donuts near us and pay for the order of the car behind us. As we drove down Route 109, it quickly turned into a fun game as he gleefully shouted from his car seat, "What's the next drive thru?!" With each stop, he kept hoping that the car behind us would do the same as we had just done for them. This chain mail of kindness led us to bigger plans as the years went on.

What my kids have taken from the Toddsgiving experience is a knowledge that we can feel all the feelings at once. We talk throughout the year about feeling "smad" (sad and mad) or feeling "nervcited" (nervous and excited). They know that on November 19, we can feel "prad"—proud of how we are honoring Todd's spirit and sad that more memories aren't being made with Todd. It has become the way my kids now think about loss and think about challenges in life—we can be mad, sad, proud, smad, and prad all at once as we find ways to bring that spirit to anyone who needs it.

Coaching Tweens Through the Interference

Coaching kids toward kindness can feel trickier when they hit adolescence. Your tween may suddenly seem allergic to your advice. Phyllis Fagell is a school counselor, psychotherapist, and author of *Middle School Matters: The 10 Key Skills Kids Need to Thrive in Middle School and Beyond—and How Parents Can Help*. Basically, she is the Middle School Whisperer, and I come away inspired every time I talk with her.

For many adults, the words *middle school* evoke a negative, gut-level response. We might remember being rejected by a friend, being insecure about body changes, or being embarrassed by a teacher. That can make parenting these years extra difficult, because "you are bringing all of that to the table as your child approaches middle school," said Fagell.

It's an age of contradiction, Fagell told me. "They have an interest in taking moral action and fixing everything wrong with the world, and yet they are complicated and can create major drama in their own social lives that's inconsistent with their heightened sense of justice." Fagell offers this image to help parents reconcile why middle schoolers make poor choices: "Your child is an inherently good kid, but there will be all kinds of interference in middle school." That interference might be fear (*If I stand up for this person, will I be targeted?*). That interference might also be jealousy or insecurity. They want the approval of their peers—*and* they need the support of adults more than ever.

The inherent messiness of this stage gives parents an opportunity to "get in there and make a difference," says Fagell. "Rather than looking at this phase with dread, see it as an opportunity to share your values and solidify your relationship with your children." Middle schoolers are impressionable. Rather than stepping back, she encourages parents to lean in and practice radical curiosity. Don't let their aloofness fool you. Yes, they are biologically predisposed to seek peer approval at this age. Still, middle schoolers are also hyperaware of the adults in their lives and hungry for their love and attention.

During these years, you can capitalize on your tween's growing sense of justice to articulate an attractive vision of who they can be. Give them access to awe-inspiring stories, mentors, and activities. "Vocalize your family's values, such as, *In this family, we value kindness, and we treat each other well*," says Fagell. "Help them understand the impact they are having on others. When they hurt someone's feelings—and they will—ask, *How would you feel if someone did this to you or your sister or brother? How can you make it better? Instead of just saying sorry, how can you make amends?*"

The Awesome Power of One Caring Adult

Few things bring me more awe than watching adults help a child who is not their own. Fred Rogers and I fully agree on this. "Anyone who does anything to help a child in his life is a hero to me," he once said.[27]

The word *hero* here isn't hyperbole. Researchers at Harvard's Center for the Developing Child looked at data from thousands of children who had experienced adverse childhood experiences. They wanted to know: Why were some kids more resilient than others? Resilience is a psychological capacity that allows us to adjust and adapt to life's challenges. Resilient people keep challenges and setbacks in perspective, have strategies for navigating difficult emotions, and have the strength to bounce back and take another step forward. The researchers found that "the single most common factor for children who develop resilience is at least one stable and committed relationship with a supportive parent, caregiver, or other adult."[28]

When I talked to Lisa Damour, author of *The Emotional Life of Teenagers*, she echoed this sentiment. According to Damour, the most potent force for good in a teenager's life is a "caring, working relationship with at least one loving adult." Within that context, adults can offer teenagers empathy, grounded perspective, and a vote of confidence as they work through challenges.

Many parents will have the opportunity to be that "one adult" for a child outside of our immediate family—like a niece, a nephew, or a neighbor. And sometimes kids cross our path unexpectedly, and so increasing our ability to meet their needs is a proactive kindness. Kids, no matter their age, need multiple adults to circle up around them.

Michele Borba began her career teaching in a classroom for children with significant learning differences—differences that sometimes led to emotional challenges as they tried to navigate a school system that didn't seem built for them. As she got to know each student, one question guided Borba: How can I help them shine? This work took patience, practice, and curiosity. She paid close attention to the child in front of her—not who the school file or previous teacher *said* was in front of her. Take Rick, a first grader who "was always by my side but would never verbalize what he wanted or needed." Over time, Borba noticed him doodling on his papers. "Wow," she whispered to him one day, "you are really good at this."

"That was the first time I ever saw him smile," she told me. Later, she casually posted his work for others to see, praised his creativity to other teachers in his earshot, and helped his parents find an afterschool art club. Many years later, Borba got a letter from Rick—now a professional artist—thanking her for the day she put his picture on the bulletin board. "That was the day I stopped worrying if kids would think I was stupid," he wrote.

Borba's awe-inspiring story reminded me of an Oprah Winfrey interview with the Pulitzer Prize–winning novelist Toni Morrison.[29] Morrison described how, when her children came into the room, she thought she was showing care by fussing over their appearance "to see if they had buckled their trousers or if their hair was combed or if their socks were up." But they were looking for something else, she said. Morrison offered up a different way to show care: Does your face light up when your kid walks into a room? Does your expression say, *I'm so glad you are here*?

Does your face light up? That question became my anchor as both a parent and a teacher. Working with kids is beautifully messy work. We bump against each other and fiddle with each other's most vulnerable buttons. We don't always get it right. Morrison's words offer grace— something simple and sacred that we can do every day. When my kids come down bleary-eyed and cranky in the morning, I can give them a smile. My face can be a safe landing place when they arrive home from school. And when they go to bed at night, I can muster up a final *I love you*, even if the evening went awry.

"For four years of playing the saxophone, it was my biggest fear to mess up during a performance. Then, one night, in front of my entire school, my biggest fear came true. The piano was off a measure, my fingers fumbled, the drum stuttered, and the bassist looked up in confusion. It wasn't like my nightmares, though. No one booed. I just laughed so hard it came out of my instrument in a squawk. Our instructor, smiling, called out the measure and clapped his hands to the beat. We got back on track. At the end, we stood to bow. It was the most applause I've ever received. I hadn't realized that it was okay to mess up like that. I hadn't realized that I belonged to a community that would still support me. I was so amazed looking around at my fellow band members, each of us smiling in sheer disbelief that we had survived that. At that moment, it felt like I could do anything."
—Naomi Hopkins, high schooler

A few years ago, when searching for the Toni Morrison video clip to share with a friend, I discovered that I had gotten her quote wrong—by one word. She does not say when *your* kid walks in a room. Instead, she says, "When a kid walks in a room—your child or anybody else's child—does your face light up? That's what they're looking for . . . let your face speak what's in your heart. . . . It's just as small as that."

A kid. Anybody's child.

Morrison wasn't just talking about parenting. She was talking about our obligation to see the dignity in every person—a dignity that Mr. Rogers offered children every day when he signed off his show with, "You've made this day a special day, by just your being you. There's no person in the whole world like you, and I like you just the way you are."

My kids are watching my face in the grocery line. They watch how I greet the elderly woman in front of us and the young man behind us. They watch how I greet their friends on the playground and interact with a stranger who stops to ask for directions. They watch my comfort—or discomfort—in interacting with people with different temperaments and abilities. They are looking for clues. Does my face light up still?

A Final Thought

I still love checking in on my friend Rachel's Tiny Kindness project. I have not read every post over the years—she's posted thousands of them—but in December 2021, I clicked on her feed and saw this.

> My fifth-grade teacher gave me a little note of encouragement one day when I was struggling. When I got a traumatic brain injury from an abusive relationship in college that caused serious side effects, I pinned the note up and read it every day. Ms. Kris's kindness in fifth grade is helping me heal over ten years later.
> —name withheld, Summit, New Jersey

Wait, what? I am a "Ms. Kris." I taught fifth grade in Summit, New Jersey, during that period. What are the chances . . .?

I had no idea which student this was, much less what I had written on that little note. Rachel passed along my contact info to this anonymous former student—who had no idea that Rachel and I knew each other—just in case she wanted to reconnect. She did. We did. This amazing young woman shared her story of strength and healing with me. I reaffirmed the lasting sentiment of that tiny note all those years ago.

How did this happen? Why did she stumble upon my friend's project and submit a story? Why did I happen to read it? It's an exquisite mystery that's beyond my understanding. It is the very definition of awe.

20 Wonderful Ways
to Spread Kindness with Kids

1. Clean up a mess you didn't make.

2. Leave a kind note or drawing on a family member's pillow.

3. Pick up trash around the neighborhood.

4. Make a thank-you card for a community helper.

5. Pay someone a compliment.

6. Invite someone new to sit with you at lunch or to play with you at recess.

7. Notice when a classmate looks sad and say something kind.

8. Leave a surprise—flowers, homemade cookies, or a kindness rock—on a neighbor's doorstep.

9. Collect items to drop off at a local food pantry or animal shelter.

10. Clean and beautify a spot in the house without being asked.

11. Make cards to send to a senior center or veterans home.

12. Help rake a neighbor's leaves or clean up their yard after a storm.

13. Read a story to someone younger than you.

14. Make a family member's bed.

15. Think of a way to help your teacher and do it.

16. Tell someone that you love them.

17. Make a bird feeder or plant bulbs for spring flowers.

18. Help your parent make dinner.

19. Make a get-well card for someone.

20. Record a happy song or dance and send it to someone who needs a pick-me-up.

10 Awe-Inspiring Picture Books About Human Goodness

Last Stop on Market Street **by Matt de la Peña and Christian Robinson.** This award-winning book follows a boy and his grandmother as they take a public bus across town. His grandmother's interest in and compassion for the people they encounter on their trip leaves a lasting impression on her grandson—and the reader.

Good People Everywhere **by Lynea Gillen and Kristina Swarner.** This book echoes Fred Rogers's famous advice during times of tragedy, "Look for the helpers," and describes ordinary people in our communities doing good things—from farmers to doctors to teachers to builders.

Harlem Grown: How One Big Idea Transformed a Neighborhood **by Tony Hillery and Jessie Hartland.** This book tells the true story of Harlem Grown, a New York City garden project. This garden was once an abandoned lot, and now it helps feed the neighborhood.

Something Good **by Marcy Campbell and Corinna Luyken.** "Something bad" was written on a wall at an elementary school, and it changes the tone of the community. With time and communication, the kids and adults come together to create "something good."

Somebody Loves You, Mr. Hatch **by Eileen Spinelli and Paul Yalowitz.** On a wintry day, a lonely man named Mr. Hatch gets an unexpected package in the mail, wrapped in a big pink bow with the words "Somebody loves you." These three words transform him and lead to some unexpected surprises.

The Big Umbrella **by Amy June Bates and Juniper Bates.** Written by a mother-daughter pair, this book is told from the perspective of a helpful umbrella that somehow can make room for absolutely everyone.

Be Kind **by Pat Zietlow Miller and Jen Hill.** When Tanisha spills grape juice all over her new dress, her classmate wants to make her feel better, wondering: *What does it mean to be kind?* The rest of the book ponders this question in concrete ways.

Have You Filled a Bucket Today? **by Carol McCloud and David Messing.** "All day long, everyone in the world walks around carrying an invisible bucket . . . You feel happy and good when your bucket is full, and you feel sad and lonely when your bucket is empty." Using this simple metaphor, the author encourages children to be "bucket fillers" by showing kindness and love to others.

Each Kindness **by Jacqueline Woodson and E. B. Lewis.** In this award-winning book, a child name Chloe reflects on the way she and her friends excluded a new student. She begins to wonder how things would be different if she had chosen compassion and inclusion.

A Chair for My Mother **by Vera B. Williams.** After their belongings are destroyed in a fire, a grandmother, mother, and young daughter save up for a soft chair for snuggling and resting at the end of the day. The family is helped along the way by kind neighbors, relatives, and coworkers—highlighting the importance of extending love and support to those in need.

AFTERWORD

The news: everything is bad.
Poets: okay, but what if everything is bad and we still fall in love
with the moon and learn something from the flowers.

—Nikita Gill

In recounting some of the struggles she faced in her life, poet Mary Oliver once said, "I got saved by the beauty of the world."[1] Nature, music, art, big questions, belonging, the circle of life, human kindness—we walk in and through such beauty every day. And yet it can still feel so unexpected when awe strikes.

Anna, a high schooler, told me that she feels awe in moments of surprise: "A surprisingly beautiful flower on what I assumed to be a mundane walk to the train. A surprisingly warm smile in a strained friendship. A surprisingly meaningful conversation when I thought things would be awkward. A surprising act of kindness on a day when I felt like there was no more goodness in the world."

When I stumbled upon the trove of awe research in 2021, I had no idea it would take me on a personal, professional, and parenting journey. It's not that this research has radically changed my life—at least not in ways that would be visible to others. Instead, it has taken my ordinary life and made it richer. Perhaps that is radical.

Seeking awe has been like getting the piano tuned or putting on the right prescription glasses: The sounds are more resonant, the images clearer. I have become more grounded in this world and its simple wonders, more apt to notice my kids' laughter in the car, take a mental snapshot during a family walk, look for small kindnesses, and share what I find with others. Awe-seeking has become a way of seeing, and in this busy, scary, messy business of raising kids, awe has made me more attuned to the things that matter most.

Take last night.

I took my son to a Red Sox game at Fenway Park. A thunderstorm was just clearing, and sunbeams shot through gray clouds. As we waited to get in, he pointed out the bricked-in "Fenway Park 1912" sign, flanked by World Series banners. As we found our seats, I noticed the Jimmy Fund Cancer Research wall display, and we hunted for a picture of his friend's Uncle Todd (who you read about in chapter 7), a Red Sox fan and Jimmy Fund ambassador who died of cancer at age nineteen.

Once seated, I saw the #42 posted in the rafters. That's Jackie Robinson's number. My sports-fact-loving child informed me that the league retired this number for *all* MLB teams in 1997—the first athlete honored this way in any US professional league. And because we were there on Juneteenth, the woman singing the National Anthem first graced the crowd with a soul-stirring rendition of "Lift Every Voice and Sing"—a hymn commonly known as the Black National Anthem, which includes these lines:

> Sing a song full of the faith that the dark past has taught us,
> Sing a song full of the hope that the present has brought us;
> Facing the rising sun of our new day begun,
> Let us march on 'til victory is won.

Then, in the eighth inning, we joined 33,000 other Red Sox fans in belting out "Sweet Caroline," a quirky, beloved Fenway Park tradition. And later, as we returned to the car, my kid—filled with excitement and a bit too much popcorn and nachos—suddenly vomited into the bushes on a dark Boston side street. A family passed us with a look of sympathy. But a minute later the mom came racing back and pressed some napkins into my hand. "I've been there," she said.

Yes, I'm a little tired this morning, but I'm also filled with intense gratitude for that evening with my kid. An evening made that much richer because we took time to notice and talk about:

1. The brooding sky (Nature)

2. The beauty of "Lift Every Voice and Sing" (Music)

3. The architectural details of Fenway Park (Art)

4. The meaning of #42 and Juneteenth (Big Questions)

5. The Jimmy Fund Cancer Research poster (The Circle of Life)

6. The experience of singing and cheering in harmony with 33,000 people (Belonging)

7. The stranger who saw a need, filled it, and then disappeared back into the night (Human Kindness)

The evening was made more meaningful and memorable because I sought and found awe, and I was able to share that feeling with my amazing kid.

That's my hope in writing this book—that we will help our kids experience this powerful emotion by raising them to be awe-seekers and by becoming awe-seekers ourselves.

ACKNOWLEDGMENTS

The most common source of awe is human goodness, and I get goosebumps when I think of the good people who helped make this book a reality.

First, thank you to Dacher Keltner, whose rich research inspired this entire project and whose book *Awe: The New Science of Everyday Wonder and How It Can Transform Your Life* is a must-read. When I interviewed you in 2021 for that *Washington Post* article, I off-handedly mentioned that I wished there were a parenting book about this subject. You replied, "Maybe that's your book to write." I guess it was.

My deep gratitude to all the kids, teens, parents, researchers, and educators—nearly seventy of you!—who said "yes" when I asked for your insights about awe and wonder. This would not be a book without your words and your wisdom. Special thanks to the schools that allowed me to visit and/or speak with their students and teachers, including The Rashi School, Montrose School, Riverbend School, Brilla Public Charter Schools, Medfield Children's Center, and Kent Place.

I am so lucky to have landed at Free Spirit Publishing. Kyra Ostendorf, Amanda Shofner, Tom Rademacher, and Cassie Labriola-Sitzman have not only championed this endeavor (and all my other books), but they are also some of the kindest people you could ever hope to know. Tom, you knew this was the book I *really* wanted to write, even though I pitched you a different one. Cassie, you are a brilliant *and* gentle editor, and you nurtured this project with such care. Emily Bond, having you on my team makes everything better.

Thank you to Mary Hope Garcia at PBS KIDS and Ki Sung at KQED's *MindShift* for inviting me to write about child development on these platforms for the last decade. This work has helped shape my voice and given me access to remarkable thinkers and researchers.

A special shout-out to Charles River Coffee House for letting me spend hours working away at that table by the window. Your lattes and playlists played a material part in getting this book done. I'm also so lucky to have two independent bookstores near me—Wellesley Books and Aesop's Books—who have provided the kind of support that authors dream about.

I'm forever grateful for my village: the friends who live close enough to hug and the friends who lift me up from a distance; our neighborhood, one of those special places "where everybody knows your name"; the group of moms whom I regularly text about all the small victories, big worries, and everyday wonders of raising young humans; all the teachers who have showered my kids with support; my beautiful mom and four older siblings who raised me and (still!) love and support me.

Boundless gratitude to my dad: while you didn't get to meet my kids, your radical curiosity about, well, *everything* is very much alive in them. Your fingerprints are all over this book.

Michael, Aster, and James: you are my greatest source of awe. You are my everything. You also explicitly told me to give the final shout-out to Cupid, our wonder pup. So there you go.

NOTES

Introduction

Epigraph. Dacher Keltner, *Awe: The New Science of Everyday Wonder and How It Can Transform Your Life* (Penguin Random House, 2023), 229.

1. Summer Allen, "The Science of Awe," white paper, prepared for the John Templeton Foundation by the Greater Good Science Center at UC Berkeley (September 2018), ggsc.berkeley.edu/images/uploads/GGSC-JTF_White_Paper-Awe_FINAL.pdf.; Deborah Farmer Kris, "Awe Might Be Our Most Undervalued Emotion. Here's How to Help Children Find It," *Washington Post*, November 30, 2021, washingtonpost.com/lifestyle/on-parenting/children-awe-emotion/2021/11/29/0f78a4b0-4c8e-11ec-b0b0-766bbbe79347_story.html.

2. Dacher Keltner, *Awe: The New Science of Everyday Wonder and How It Can Transform Your Life* (Penguin Random House, 2023), XXV, 42–44.

3. Keltner, *Awe*, 26.

4. Allen, "The Science of Awe."

5. Craig Anderson, Maria Monroy, and Dacher Keltner, "Awe in Nature Heals: Evidence from Military Veterans, At-Risk Youth, and College Students," *Emotion* 18, no. 8 (December 2018): 1195–1202, doi.org/10.1037/emo0000442.

6. Craig Anderson, Dante Dixson, Maria Monroy, and Dacher Keltner, "Are Awe-Prone People More Curious? The Relationship Between Dispositional Awe, Curiosity, and Academic Outcomes," *Journal of Personality* 88, no. 4 (November 2019): 762–779, doi.org/10.1111/jopy.12524.

7. Keltner, *Awe*, 230.

8. Dacher Keltner, "Why Do We Feel Awe?" *Greater Good Magazine*, May 10, 2016, greatergood.berkeley.edu/article/item/why_do_we_feel_awe.

9. Artemisia O'bi and Fan Yang, "Self-Transcendent Experiences Early in Life: Children Appreciate Diverse Effects of Awe-Inspiring Experiences" (February 2023): 32, doi.org/10.31234/osf.io/72x3y.

10. Dacher Keltner, "What's the Most Common Source of Awe?" *Greater Good Magazine*, January 24, 2023, greatergood.berkeley.edu/article/item/whats_the_most_common_source_of_awe.

11. Challenge Success, "'PDF' Tips," May 14, 2021, challengesuccess.org/resources/pdf-tips/.

12. Deborah Farmer Kris, "Three Things Overscheduled Kids Need More of in Their Lives," *MindShift*, August 26, 2019, kqed.org/mindshift/54248/three-things-overscheduled-kids-need-more-of-in-their-lives.

13. Robert Waldinger and Marc Schulz, *The Good Life: Lessons from the World's Longest Scientific Study of Happiness* (Simon and Schuster, 2023).; Deborah Farmer Kris, "The Mundane, Radical, Fun, Painful Ways We Can Help Our Kids Find Happiness," *Washington Post*, January 19, 2023, washingtonpost.com/parenting/2023/01/17/happy-kids-research-good-life.

Chapter 1: The Wonder of Nature

Epigraph. Rachel Carson, *The Sense of Wonder: A Celebration of Nature for Parents and Children* (Harper Collins, 1998), 54.

1. Christopher Maag, "A Divided America Agrees on One Thing: The Eclipse Was Awesome," *New York Times*, April 9, 2024, nytimes.com/2024/04/09/nyregion/total-solar-eclipse.html.

2. Deborah Farmer Kris, "How to Watch the Solar Eclipse with Your Kids," *PBS KIDS*, April 5, 2024, pbs.org/parents/thrive/how-to-watch-the-solar-eclipse-with-your-kids.

3. Richard Louv, *Last Child in the Woods: Saving Our Children from Nature-Deficit Disorder* (Algonquin Books, 2008).; Danielle Cohen, "Why Kids Need to Spend Time in Nature," Child Mind Institute, updated October 30, 2023, childmind.org/article/why-kids-need-to-spend-time-in-nature.; Amber Fyfe-Johnson, Marnie F. Hazlehurst, Sara P. Perrins, Gregory N. Bratman, Rick Thomas, Kimberly A. Garrett, Kiana R. Hafferty, Tess M. Cullaz, Edgar K. Marcuse, and Pooja S. Tandon, "Nature and Children's Health: A Systematic Review," *Pediatrics* 148, no. 4 (October 2021): e2020049155, doi.org/10.1542/peds.2020-049155.

4. Chih-Da Wu, Eileen McNeely, J. G. Cedeño-Laurent, Wen-Chi Pan, Gary Adamkiewicz, Francesca Dominici, Shih-Chun Candice Lung, Huey-Jen Su, and John D. Spengler, "Linking Student Performance in Massachusetts Elementary Schools with the 'Greenness' of School Surroundings Using Remote Sensing," *PLOS ONE* 9, no. 10 (October 2014): e108548, doi.org/10.1371/journal.pone.0108548.

5. Victoria Rideout, Alanna Peebles, Supreet Mann, and Michael Robb, *The Common Sense Census: Media Use by Tweens and Teens, 2021* (Common Sense, 2022), commonsensemedia.org/sites/default/files/research/report/8-18-census-integrated-report-final-web_0.pdf.

6. SGB Media, "Kamik Survey: Children Spending 35 Percent Less Time Playing Freely Outside," September 20, 2018, sgbonline.com/kamik-survey-childre-spending-35-percent-less-time-playing-freely-outside.

7. Dacher Keltner, *Awe: The New Science of Everyday Wonder and How It Can Transform Your Life* (Penguin Random House, 2023), 128.

8. Yang Bai, Joseph Ocampo, Gening Jin, Serena Chen, Veronica Benet-Martinez, Maria Monroy, Craig Anderson, and Dacher Keltner, "Awe, Daily Stress, and Elevated Life Satisfaction," *Journal of Personality and Social Psychology* 120, no. 4 (April 2021): 837–860, doi.org/10.1037/pspa0000267.

9. Craig Anderson, Maria Monroy, and Dacher Keltner, "Awe in Nature Heals: Evidence from Military Veterans, At-Risk Youth, and College Students," *Emotion* 18, no. 8 (December 2018): 1195–1202, doi.org/10.1037/emo0000442.

10. UC Berkeley, "A Veteran's Journey into Nature Reduced his PTSD," Video, filmed by Roxanne Makasdjian and Stephen McNally, posted May 31, 2016, YouTube, 5:15, youtube.com/watch?v=hIjK-9hOOIY.

11. Anderson, Monroy, and Keltner, "Awe in Nature Heals."

12. Jill Suttie, "Why Is Nature So Good for Your Mental Health?" *Greater Good Magazine*, April 19, 2019, greatergood.berkeley.edu/article/item/why_is_nature_so_good_for_your_mental_health.

13. Kirsten Beyer, Andrea Kaltenbach, Aniko Szabo, Sandra Bogar, F. Javier Nieto, and Kristen M. Malecki, "Exposure to Neighborhood Green Space and Mental Health: Evidence from the Survey of the Health of Wisconsin," *International Journal of Environmental Research and Public Health* 11, no. 3 (March 2014): 3453–3472, doi.org/10.3390/ijerph110303453.

14. Nancy Wells, "At Home with Nature: Effects of, 'Greenness,' on Children's Cognitive Functioning," *Environment and Behavior* 32, no. 6 (November 2000): 775–795, doi.org/10.1177/00139160021972793.

15. Nissa Towe-Goodman, et al., "Green Space and Internalizing or Externalizing Symptoms Among Children," *JAMA Network Open* 7, no. 4 (April 2024): e245742, doi.org/10.1001/jamanetworkopen.2024.5742.

16. Brian Doctrow, "Green Space May Improve Young Children's Mental Health," *NIH Research Matters*, April 30, 2024, nih.gov/news-events/nih-research-matters/green-space-may-improve-young-children-s-mental-health.

17. Paul Piff, Pia Dietze, Matthew F. Feinberg, Daniel M. Stancato, and Dacher Keltner, "Awe, the Small Self, and Prosocial Behavior," *Journal of Personality and Social Psychology* 108, no. 6 (2015): 883–899, dx.doi.org/10.1037/pspi0000018.

18. Adam Hoffman, "How Awe Makes Us Generous," *Greater Good Magazine*, August 3, 2015, greatergood.berkeley.edu/article/item/how_awe_makes_us_generous.

19. Piff et al., "Awe, the Small Self, and Prosocial Behavior."

20. Ethan Kross, *Chatter: The Voice in Our Heads, Why It Matters, and How to Harness It* (Crown, 2021).

21. Rachel Carson, *The Sense of Wonder: A Celebration of Nature for Parents and Children* (Harper Collins, 1998), 69.

22. Virginia E. Sturm et al., "Big Smile, Small Self: Awe Walks Promote Prosocial Positive Emotions in Older Adults," *Emotion* 22, no. 5 (August 2022): 1044–1058, doi.org/10.1037/emo0000876.

23. Aran Levasseur, "How Awe Walks Helped My Students Slow Down," *Greater Good Magazine*, September 8, 2023, greatergood.berkeley.edu/article/item/how_awe_walks_helped_my_students_slow_down.

24. Qing Li, "Effects of Forest Environment (Shinrin-yoku/Forest bathing) on Health Promotion and Disease Prevention—the Establishment of 'Forest Medicine,'" *Environmental Health and Preventative Medicine* 27 (November 2022): 43, doi.org/ 10.1265/ehpm.22-00160.

25. Vicki Thomas, "Fascinated by Nature," film by Reflections of Life, November 15, 2017, 3:27, grateful.org/resource/fascinated-by-nature.

26. Thomas, "Fascinated by Nature."

27. Stephen Kaplan, "The Restorative Benefits of Nature: Toward an Integrative Framework," *Journal of Environmental Psychology* 15 (1995): 169–182, doi.org/10.1016/0272-4944(95)90001-2.

28. Annie Murphy Paul, *The Extended Mind: The Power of Thinking Outside the Brain* (Houghton Miflin Harcourt, 2021).

29. Marily Oppezzo and Daniel Schwartz, "Give Your Idea Some Legs: The Positive Effect of Walking on Creative Thinking," *Journal of Experimental Psychology* 40, no. 4 (July 2014): 1142–1152, doi.org/10.1037/a0036577.

30. Deborah Farmer Kris, "How Movement and Exercise Help Kids Learn," *MindShift*, May 21, 2019, kqed.org/mindshift/53681/how-movement-and-exercise-help-kids-learn.

31. Maria Montessori, *From Childhood to Adolescence*, The Montessori Series, vol. 12 (Montessori-Pierson Publishing, 2007), 19.

Chapter 2: The Wonder of Music

Epigraph. Phil Roura, "Moving Spirit: Mary J. Blige Is on a Soul-Stirring Crusade While on Tour," *New York Daily News*, October 2, 2010, nydailynews.com/2010/10/02/moving-spirit-mary-j-blige-is-on-a-soul-stirring-crusade-while-on-tour.

1. Eftychia Stamkou, Eddie Brummelman, Rohan Dunham, Milica Nikolic, and Dacher Keltner, "Awe Sparks Prosociality in Children," *Psychological Science* 34, no. 4 (February 2023): 455–467, doi.org/10.1177/09567976221150616.

2. Tracy McKay, Twitter reply to Yo-YoMa (@YoYo_Ma), "In these days of anxiety, I wanted to find a way to continue to share some of the music that gives me comfort. The first of my #SongsOfComfort: Dvořák – 'Going Home' Stay safe." Twitter (now X), March 13, 2020, x.com/YoYo_Ma/status/1238572657278431234.

3. Marla Paul, "Music Helps Patients with Dementia Connect with Loved Ones," *Northwestern Now*, August 29, 2022, news.northwestern.edu/stories/2022/08/music-helps-patients-with-dementia-connect-with-loved-ones.

4. Rob Stein, "These Scientists Explain the Power of Music to Spark Awe," *NPR*, July 29, 2023, npr.org/sections/health-shots/2023/07/29/1190374074/these-scientists-explain-the-power-of-music-to-spark-awe.

5. Denise Winterman, "The Surprising Uses for Birdsong," *BBC News*, May 8, 2013, bbc.com/news/magazine-22298779.

6. Danielle Ferraro, Zachary D. Miller, Lauren A. Ferguson, B. Derrick Taff, Jesse R. Barber, Peter Newman, and Clinton D. Francis, "The Phantom Chorus: Birdsong Boosts Human Well-Being in Protected Areas," *Biological Sciences* 23 (December 2020), doi.org/10.1098/rspb.2020.1811.; Jessica Claris Fisher, Katherine Nesbitt Irvine, Jake Emmerson Bicknell, William Michael Hayes, Damian Fernandes, Jayalaxshmi Mistry, and Zoe Georgina Davies, "Perceived Biodiversity, Sound, Naturalness and Safety Enhance the Restorative Quality and Wellbeing Benefits of Green and Blue Space in a Neotropical City," *Science of the Total Environment* 755, no. 2 (February 2021): 143095, doi.org/10.1016/j.scitotenv.2020.143095.; Eleanor Ratcliffe, "Sound and Soundscape in Restorative Natural Environments: A Narrative Literature Review," *Frontiers in Psychology* 12 (April 2021), doi.org/10.3389/fpsyg.2021.570563.

7. Suzanne Garfinkle-Crowell, "Taylor Swift Has Rocked My Psychiatric Practice," *New York Times*, June 17, 2023, nytimes.com/2023/06/17/opinion/taylor-swift-mental-health.html.

8. Raymond Leone, "Music Can Serve as Therapy. Here's How It Can Help Reduce Anxiety." *Washington Post*, August 25, 2023, washingtonpost.com/wellness/2023/08/25/music-therapy-reduce-anxiety-strategies.

9. David Snead, "Do You Know the 'Wow' Child?," email, as published by WCRB, May 7, 2019, classicalwcrb.org/blog/2019-05-07/a-priceless-wow-moment-in-the-concert-hall.

10. Brooke Hauser, "Remember the Boy Who Said 'Wow' at Symphony Hall? Now He's 14, and There's a Picture Book About Him," *Boston Globe*, April 10, 2024, bostonglobe.com/2024/04/10/arts/remember-boy-who-said-wow-symphony-hall-now-hes-14-theres-picture-book-about-him.

11. Dan + Claudia Zanes, "Sensory Friendly," accessed October 22, 2024, danandclaudia.com/sensory-friendly.

12. Dan + Claudia Zanes, "Sensory Friendly."

Chapter 3: The Wonder of Art

Epigraph. Interview with *The Guardian*, "Julie Mehretu Paints Chaos with Chaos—from Tahrir Square to Zuccotti Park," June 20, 2013, theguardian.com/artanddesign/2013/jun/20/painting-art.

1. Jill Barshay, "PROOF POINTS: The Lesson the Arts Teach," *Hechinger Report*, January 2, 2023, hechingerreport.org/proof-points-the-lesson-the-arts-teach.

2. Daniel H. Bowen and Brian Kisida, "Investigating the Causal Effects of Arts Education," *Journal of Policy Analysis and Management* 42, no. 3 (June 2023): 624–647, doi.org/10.1002/pam.22449.

3. Rebecca Chamberlain, I. Chris McManus, Nicola Brunswick, Qona Rankin, Howard Riley, and Ryota Kanai, "Drawing on the Right Side of the Brain: A Voxel-Based Morphometry Analysis of Observational Drawing," *NeuroImage* 96 (August 2014): 167–173, doi.org/10.1016/j.neuroimage.2014.03.062.

4. Melissa Hogenboom, "Artists 'Have Structurally Different Brains,'" *BBC News*, April 17, 2014, bbc.com/news/science-environment-26925271.

5. Sheryl A. Sorby, "Educational Research in Developing 3-D Spatial Skills for Engineering Students," *International Journal of Science Education* 31, no. 3 (February 2009): 459–480, doi.org/10.1080/09500690802595839.

6. Susan Magsamen and Ivy Ross, *Your Brain on Art: How the Arts Transform Us* (Random House, 2023).

7. Heather Stuckey and Jeremy Nobel, "The Connection Between Art, Healing, and Public Health: A Review of Current Literature," *American Journal of Public Health* 100, no. 2 (February 2010): 254–263, doi.org/10.2105/AJPH.2008.156497.

8. Senhu Wang, Hei Wan Mak, and Daisy Fancourt, "Arts, Mental Distress, Mental Health Functioning, and Life Satisfaction: Fixed-Effects Analyses of a Nationally-Representative Panel Study," *BMC Public Health* 20 (February 2020), 208, doi.org/10.1186/s12889-019-8109-y.

9. Akiho Sugita, Ling Ling, Taishi Tsuji, Katsunori Kondo, and Ichiro Kawachi, "Cultural Engagement and Incidence of Cognitive Impairment: A 6-year Longitudinal Follow-up of the Japan Gerontological Evaluation Study (JAGES)," *Journal of Epidemiology* 31, no. 10 (October 2021): 545–553, doi.org/10.2188/jea.JE20190337.

10. Eleanor Brown, Mallory L. Garnett, Kate E. Anderson, and Jean-Philippe Laurenceau, "Can the Arts Get Under the Skin? Arts and Cortisol for Economically Disadvantaged Children," *Child Development* 88, no. 4 (2017): 1368–1381, doi.org/10.1111/cdev.12652.

11. Clancy Blair and C. Cybele Raver, "Poverty, Stress, and Brain Development: New Directions for Prevention and Intervention," *Academic Pediatrics* 16, no. 3 (2016): 0– 6, doi.org/10.1016/j.acap.2016.01.010.

12. Dacher Keltner, *Awe: The New Science of Everyday Wonder and How It Can Transform Your Life* (Penguin Random House, 2023).

13. Project Zero, "See, Think, Wonder: A Thinking Routine from Project Zero, Harvard Graduate School of Education" (Harvard University, 2022), pz.harvard.edu/sites/default/files/See%20Think%20Wonder_3.pdf.

Chapter 4: The Wonder of Big Questions

Epigraph. Stephen Hawking, interview by Larry King, *Larry King Live*, CNN, December 25, 1999.

1. Emma Elsworthy, "Curious Children Ask 73 Questions Each Day— Many of Which Parents Can't Answer, Says Study," *Independent*, December 3, 2017, independent.co.uk/news/uk/home-news/curious-children-questions-parenting-mum-dad-google-answers-inquisitive-argos-toddlers-chad-valley-tots-town-a8089821.html.

2. Summer Allen, "The Science of Awe," white paper, prepared for the John Templeton Foundation by the Greater Good Science Center at UC Berkeley (September 2018), ggsc.berkeley.edu/images/uploads/GGSC-JTF_White_Paper-Awe_FINAL.pdf.

3. Craig Anderson, Dante Dixson, Maria Monroy, and Dacher Keltner, "Are Awe-Prone People More Curious? The Relationship Between Dispositional Awe, Curiosity, and Academic Outcomes," *Journal of Personality* 88, no. 4 (November 2019): 762–779, doi.org/10.1111/jopy.12524.

4. Paul Silvia, "Knowledge Emotions: Feelings That Foster Learning, Exploring, and Reflecting," in R. Biswas-Diener and E. Diener (eds,), *Noba Textbook Series: Psychology* (DEF Publishers, 2024), http://noba.to/f7rvqp54.

5. Silvia, "Knowledge Emotions."

6. Matthias Gruber and Charan Ranganath, "How Curiosity Enhances Hippocampus-Dependent Memory: The Prediction, Appraisal, Curiosity, and Exploration (PACE) Framework," *Trends in Cognitive Sciences* 23, no. 12 (2019): 1014–1025, doi.org/10.1016/j.tics.2019.10.003.

7. Matthias Gruber, Bernard Gelman, and Charan Ranganath, "States of Curiosity Modulate Hippocampus-Dependent Learning via the Dopaminergic Circuit," *Neuron* 84, no. 2 (October 2014): 486–496, doi.org/10.1016/j. neuron.2014.08.060.

8. Andy Fell, "Curiosity Helps Learning and Memory," University of California, Davis, October 2, 2014, universityofcalifornia.edu/news/ curiosity-helps-learning-and-memory.

9. Alice Chirico,Vlad Petre Glaveanu, Pietro Cipresso, Giuseppe Riva, and Andrea Gaggioli, "Awe Enhances Creative Thinking: An Experimental Study, " *Creativity Research Journal* 30, no. 2 (April 2018), 123–131, doi.org/1 0.1080/10400419.2018.1446491.; Jia Wei Zhang et al., "Awe Is Associated with Creative Personality, Convergent Creativity, and Everyday Creativity," *Psychology of Aesthetics, Creativity, and the Arts* 18, no. 2 (April 2024): 209–221, doi.org/10.1037/aca0000442.

10. Helen De Cruz, "The Necessity of Awe," *Aeon*, July 10, 2020, aeon.co/essays/ how-awe-drives-scientists-to-make-a-leap-into-the-unknown.

11. Dacher Keltner, "Why Do We Feel Awe?" *Greater Good Magazine*, May 10, 2016, greatergood.berkeley.edu/article/item/why_do_we_feel_awe.

12. Warren Berger, *A More Beautiful Question: The Power of Inquiry to Spark Breakthrough Ideas* (Bloomsbury, 2016), 9.

13. Warren Berger, "These Three Questions Can Help You Tackle Any Problem," accessed October 22, 2024, amorebeautifulquestion.com/ three-questions-can-help-tackle-problem.

14. Bill Whitaker, host, "Teens Surprise Math World with Pythagorean Theorem Trigonometry Proof," *60 Minutes*, May 6, 2024, YouTube, 13:18, youtube.com/watch?v=VheWndnHuQs.

15. Dacher Keltner, "How Awe Leads Us to Purpose and Meaning," interview by Thomas Bernett, *Templeton Ideas*, John Templeton Foundation, audio, 29 minutes, templeton.org/news/how-awe-leads-us-to-purpose-and-meaning.

16. Robin Wall Kimmerer, *Braiding Sweetgrass: Indigenous Wisdom, Scientific Knowledge, and the Teachings of Plants* (Milkweed Editions, 2015).

17. Ben Mardell, Jen Ryan, Mara Krechevsky, Megina Baker, Savhannah Schulz, and Yvonne Liu Constant, *A Pedagogy of Play: Supporting Playful Learning in Classrooms and Schools*, (Project Zero, 2023), pz.harvard.edu/sites/default/files/PoP%20Book.pdf.

18. Rebecca J. M. Gotlieb, Xiao-Fei Yang, and Mary Helen Immordino-Yang, "Diverse Adolescents' Transcendent Thinking Predicts Young Adult Psychosocial Outcomes via Brain Network Development," *Nature: Scientific Reports* 14, no. 1 (March 2024): 6254, doi.org/10.1038/s41598-024-56800-0.

19. Xiaodong Lin-Siegler, Janet N. Ahn, Jondou Chen, Fu-Fen Anny Fan, and Myra Luna-Lucero, "Even Einstein Struggled: Effects of Learning About Great Scientists' Struggles on High School Students' Motivation to Learn Science," *Journal of Educational Psychology* 108, no. 3 (2016): 314–328, doi.org/10.1037/edu0000092.

20. NOVA, "The Science of Smart: The Power of Interest," The Secret Life of Scientists and Engineers, *PBS*, November 5, 2013, pbs.org/wgbh/nova/article/the-science-of-smart-the-power-of-interest.

21. Judith M. Harackiewicz, Jessi L. Smith, and Stacy J. Priniski, "Interest Matters: The Importance of Promoting Interest in Education," *Policy Insights from the Behavioral and Brain Sciences* 3, no. 2 (2016): 220–227, doi.org/10.1177/2372732216655542.

22. Tenelle Porter, "The Benefits of Admitting When You Don't Know," *Behavioral Scientist*, April 20, 2018, behavioralscientist.org/the-benefits-of-admitting-when-you-dont-know/.

23. Kimmerer, *Braiding Sweetgrass*.

24. Michele Borba, *Thrivers: The Surprising Reasons Why Some Kids Struggle and Others Shine* (G. P. Putnam's Sons, 2021).

25. Mihaly Csikszentmihalyi, *Flow: The Psychology of Optimal Experience* (Harper Perennial, 2008 reissue), 4.

26. Csikszentmihalyi, *Flow*, 3.

27. Benjamin Bloom, *Developing Talent in Young People* (Ballantine Books, 1985).

28. Gregg Behr and Ryan Rydzewski, *When You Wonder, You're Learning: Mister Rogers' Enduring Lessons for Raising Creative, Curious, Caring Kids* (Hachette, 2021).

Chapter 5: The Wonder of Belonging

Epigraph. Kurt Vonnegut, Jr., commencement address to the 1974 class of Hobart and William Smith Colleges, May 26, 1974, hws.edu/news/transcripts/vonnegut.aspx.

1. US Public Health Service, *Our Epidemic of Loneliness and Isolation: The U.S. Surgeon General's Advisory on the Healing Effects of Social Connection and Community* (US Public Health Service, 2023), hhs.gov/sites/default/files/surgeon-general-social-connection-advisory.pdf.

2. Ellyn Maese, "Almost a Quarter of the World Feels Lonely," *Gallup Blog*, October 24, 2023, news.gallup.com/opinion/gallup/512618/almost-quarter-world-feels-lonely.aspx.

3. APA, "New APA Poll: One in Three Americans Feels Lonely Every Week," *American Psychiatric Association*, January 30, 2024, psychiatry.org/news-room/news-releases/new-apa-poll-one-in-three-americans-feels-lonely-e.

4. Dacher Keltner, "What's the Most Common Source of Awe?" *Greater Good Magazine*, January 24, 2023, greatergood.berkeley.edu/article/item/whats_the_most_common_source_of_awe.

5. Lydia Denworth, "Brain Waves Synchronize when People Interact," *Scientific American*, July 1, 2023, scientificamerican.com/article/brain-waves-synchronize-when-people-interact.

6. Fred Rogers, *The World According to Mister Rogers: Important Things to Remember* (Hyperion, 2003).

7. KJ Dell'Antonia, "Why Kids Love a (Minor) 'Crisis,'" *New York Times*, March 14, 2014, archive.nytimes.com/parenting.blogs.nytimes.com/2014/03/14/why-kids-love-a-minor-crisis/.

8. Diana Opong, "Parents, Are You Overindulging Your Kid? This 4-Question Test Can Help You Find Out," *NPR*, September 21, 2023, npr.org/2023/09/16/1199885688/the-consequences-of-overindulging-your-kids.

9. New Victory Theater, *Spark Change: Investing in Performing Arts Education for All* (SPARK Impact Report, n.d.), newvictory.s3.amazonaws.com/Images/About/Research/spark-change-investing-in-performing-arts-education-new-42-impact-research-report.pdf.

10. Robert Waldinger and Marc Schulz, *The Good Life: Lessons from the World's Longest Scientific Study of Happiness* (Simon and Schuster, 2023), 64.

11. The Family Dinner Project, "Benefits of Family Dinners," MGH Psychiatry Academy, accessed October 22, 2024, thefamilydinnerproject.org/about-us/benefits-of-family-dinners.

12. Bruce Feiler, "The Stories That Bind Us," *New York Times*, March 17, 2013, nytimes.com/2013/03/17/fashion/the-family-stories-that-bind-us-this-life.html.

Chapter 6: The Wonder of the Circle of Life

Epigraph. Susan David, *Emotional Agility: Get Unstuck, Embrace Change, and Thrive in Work and Life* (Avery, 2016), 80.

1. Kevin Dickinson, "The 8 Wonders of Life—And How They Can Transform Yours," *Big Think*, April 3, 2023, bigthink.com/the-learning-curve/awe-the-8-wonders-of-life.

2. Maria Godoy, "Petting Other People's Dogs, Even Briefly, Can Boost Your Health," *NPR*, August 3, 2023, npr.org/sections/health shots/2023/08/03/1190728554/dog-pet-mental-health-benefits.

3. Godoy, "Petting Other People's Dogs."

4. Dickinson, "The 8 Wonders of Life."

5. Clifton Parker, "Older People Offer Resources That Children Need, Stanford Report Says," *StanfordReport*, September 8, 2016, news.stanford.edu/stories/2016/09/older-people-offer-resource-children-need-stanford-report-says.

6. Caitlynn Peetz, "A Town Put a Senior Center in Its High School, Offering a Model for an Aging Nation," *EducationWeek*, March 13, 2023, edweek.org/leadership/a-town-put-a-senior-center-in-its-high-school-offering-a-model-for-an-aging-nation/2023/03.

7. Pam Belluck, "Creating a Village to Foster a Child," *New York Times*, August 16, 2007, nytimes.com/2007/08/16/garden/16treehouse.html.

8. Fred Rogers, *You Are Special: Neighborly Words of Wisdom from Mister Rogers* (Penguin Books, 1995), chapter 8.

9. Lorna Collier, "Growth After Trauma: Why Are Some People More Resilient Than Others—And Can It Be Taught?" *Monitor on Psychology* 47, no. 10 (November 2016): 48, apa.org/monitor/2016/11/growth-trauma.

Chapter 7: The Wonder of Human Kindness

Epigraph. Maya Angelou, "Continue," in *Celebrations: Rituals of Peace and Prayer* (Random House, 2006).

1. Harvard Medical School, "Giving Thanks Can Make You Happier," Harvard Health Publishing, August 14, 2021, health.harvard.edu/healthbeat/giving-thanks-can-make-you-happier.

2. Martin E. P. Seligman, Tracy A. Steen, Nansook Park, and Christopher Peterson, "Positive Psychology Progress: Empirical Validation of Interventions," *American Psychologist* 60, no. 5 (July 2005): 410–421, doi.org/10.1037/0003-066X.60.5.410.

3. Jeffrey J. Froh, Todd B. Kashdan, Kathleen M. Ozimkowski, and Norman Miller, "Who Benefits the Most from a Gratitude Intervention in Children and Adolescents? Examining Positive Affect as a Moderator," *The Journal of Positive Psychology* 4, no. 5 (November 2008): 408–422, doi.org/10.1080/17439760902992464.

4. Dacher Keltner, "What's the Most Common Source of Awe?" *Greater Good Magazine*, January 24, 2023, greatergood.berkeley.edu/article/item/whats_the_most_common_source_of_awe.

5. Eftychia Stamkou, Eddie Brummelman, Rohan Dunham, Milica Nikolic, and Dacher Keltner, "Awe Sparks Prosociality in Children," *Psychological Science* 34, no. 4 (February 2023): 455–467, doi.org/10.1177/09567976221150616.

6. Lila Lieberman, "The Neuroscience of Compassion," *UPLIFT*, accessed October 23, 2024, uplift.love/the-neuroscience-of-compassion.

7. David R. Cregg and Jennifer S. Cheavens, "Healing Through Helping: An Experimental Investigation of Kindness, Social Activities, and Reappraisal as Well-Being Interventions," *The Journal of Positive Psychology* 18, no. 6 (December 2022): 924–941, doi.org/10.1080/17439760.2022.2154695.

8. Jeff Grabmeier, "Feeling Depressed? Performing Acts of Kindness May Help," *Ohio State News*, January 10, 2023, osu.edu/feeling-depressed-performing-acts-of-kindness-may-help.

9. Grabmeier, "Feeling Depressed?"

10. Fred Rogers, interview by Karen Herman, *Archive of American Television*, Television Academy Foundation, July 22, 1999, interviews.televisionacademy.com/interviews/fred-rogers?clip=7#interview-clips.

11. Fred Rogers, *Life's Journeys According to Mister Rogers: Things to Remember Along the Way* (Hachette, 2005).

12. Elizabeth Marks, Caroline Hickman, Panu Pihkala, Susan Clayton, Eric R. Lewandowski, Elouise E. Mayall, Britt Wray, Catriona Mellor, and Lise van Susteren "Young People's Voices on Climate Anxiety, Government Betrayal and Moral Injury: A Global Phenomenon," *The Lancet* (September 2021), dx.doi.org/10.2139/ssrn.3918955.

13. Harvard University, "Harvard Youth Poll, 2023," Harvard Kennedy School, April 24, 2023, iop.harvard.edu/youth-poll/45th-edition-spring-2023.

14. Alain Cohn, Michel André Maréchal, David Tannenbaum, and Christian Lucas Zünd, "Civic Honesty Around the Globe," *Science* 365, no. 6448 (2019): 70–73, doi.org/10.1126/science.aau8712.

15. John Green, "John Green's Reluctant Rocket Ship Ride," interview by Steven B. Levitt, *People I Mostly Admire*, podcast from Freakonomics Podcast Network, episode 92, November 11, 2022, freakonomics.com/podcast/john-greens-reluctant-rocket-ship-ride.

16. Deborah Farmer Kris, "Raising Grateful Kids: Why Giving Thanks Is Good for the Soul," *PBS KIDS*, August 22, 2016, pbs.org/parents/thrive/raising-grateful-kids-why-giving-thanks-is-good-for-the-soul.

17. KJ Dell'Antonia, *How to Be a Happier Parent: Raising a Family, Having a Life, and Loving (Almost) Every Minute* (Avery, 2018).

18. Kyle Benson, "The Magic Relationship Ratio, According to Science," The Gottman Institute, June 26, 2024, gottman.com/blog/the-magic-relationship-ratio-according-science.

19. Rachel Hunt, Tiny Kindness, tinykindness.org.

20. Rachel Hunt, Tiny Kindness.

21. Fred Rogers, *The World According to Mister Rogers: Important Things to Remember* (Hyperion, 2003).

22. Lane Beckes, James A. Coan, and Karen Hasselmo, "Familiarity Promotes the Blurring of Self and Other in the Neural Representation of Threat," *Social Cognitive and Affective Neuroscience* 8, no 6 (August 2013): 670–677, doi.org/10.1093/scan/nss046.

23. Susan Cain, *Bittersweet: How Sorrow and Longing Make Us Whole* (Crown, 2023), 97.

24. Deborah Farmer Kris, "Expanding Your Child's Circle of Concern," *PBS KIDS for Parents*, December 14, 2015, pbs.org/parents/thrive/expanding-your-childs-circle-of-concern.

25. Kevin Lanza, Ethan T. Hunt, Dale S. Mantey, Onyinye Omega-Njemnobi, Benjamin Cristol, and Steven H. Kelder, "Volunteering, Health, and Well-being of Children and Adolescents in the United States" *JAMA Network Open* 6, no. 5 (2023), doi.org/10.1001/jamanetworkopen.2023.15980.

26. Stevie N. Grassetti, Julie A. Hubbard, Marissa A. Smith, Megan K. Bookhout, Lauren E. Swift, and Michael J. Gawrysiak, "Caregivers' Advice and Children's Bystander Behaviors During Bullying Incidents," *Journal of Clinical Child and Adolescent Psychology* 47, supplement 1 (2018): 29– 40, doi.org/10.108 0/15374416.2017.1295381.

27. Rogers, *The World According to Mister Rogers*.

28. Harvard University, "Resilience," Harvard University Center on the Developing Child, accessed October 23, 2024, developingchild.harvard.edu/science/key-concepts/resilience.

29. Toni Morrison, "Toni Morrison: Does Your Face Light Up?" interview by Oprah Winfrey, *The Oprah Winfrey Show*, OWN, video clip 1:03, May 20, 2014, youtube.com/watch?v=4iIigAgDp2Q.

Afterword

Epigraph. Nikita Gill (@nktgill), "The news: everything is bad. Poets: okay, but what if everything is bad and we still fall in love with the moon and learn something from the flowers," Twitter (now X), July 12, 2022.

1. Mary Oliver, "Mary Oliver: 'I Got Saved by the Beauty of the World,'" interview by Krista Tippett, *On Being with Krista Tippett* (podcast), February 5, 2015, onbeing.org/programs/mary-oliver-i-got-saved-by-the-beauty-of-the-world.

INDEX

A

Ada's Violin (Hood and Comport), 140
Adnan, Etel, 65
The AfterGrief (Edelman), 154
Alder Hey Children's Hospital (Liverpool, England), 49
Al-Hathloul, Lina, 112
All of Us (Erskine and Boiger), 140
Allen, Summer, 89
American Psychiatric Association (APA)
Monitor on Psychology article on Tedeschi, 157
poll on loneliness, 115
Anderson, Craig, 20–21, 36
Angelou, Maya, 167
Anna at the Art Museum (Hutchins, Herbert, and Crump), 84
Apart, Together (Sweeney and Rutland), 139
art
    being an awesome art critic, 78
    benefits of for kids, 67–68, 71
    and the developing brain, 68
    going to see some art, 78–81
    and mental health, 70–72
    picture books about, 84–85
    as source of awe, 9–10
    and spatial reasoning, 68–70
    unleashing kids' inner artists, 72–77
    ways to help your kids experience art, 83–84
Arts and Learning (Harvard Graduate School of Education), 74
arts funding, for schools, 67–68
attention
    defined, 30
    nature and, 29–32
attention restoration theory (ART), 31
awe
    author's research on, 3
    and creative thinking, 93
    defined, 4–5
    healing powers of, 156
    how kids understand awe, 7–8
    importance of, 5–6
    and intellectual humility, 103–104
    as knowledge emotion, 89
    as powerful educational tool, 90
    as self-transcendent emotion, 116
    sources of, 9–10
Awe (Keltner), 6–7, 145
awe walks, 27–28
awe-curiosity connection, 89–90

B

Bai, Yang, 9
Barnett, Mac, 112
Barshay, Jill, 67–68
Basquiat, Jean-Michel, 85
Bates, Amy June, 84–85, 193
Bates, Juniper, 193
Batori, Susan, 62
Be Kind (Miller and Hill), 193
Because (Willems and Ren), 62
Because of an Acorn (Schaefer, Schaefer, and Preston-Gannon), 40
becoming awe-seeker yourself (parenting anchor), 14
Bednarski, Susan, 84
Beeke, Tiphanie, 163–164
Behr, Gregg, 90
belonging
    collective neuroscience, 116–117
    defined, 118
    kids as wanting to belong, 117–119
    learning from coaches, 125–130
    as looking different for tweens and teens, 121–123
    needing to be needed, 119–121
    and the performing arts, 130–133

picture books about, 139–140

rituals, routines, and rich connections, 134–135

ways to help your child experience belonging, 138–139

when kids struggle to fit in, 123–125

Berger, Warren, 93

big ideas

example of, 102

picture books to inspire big ideas, 111–113

as source of awe, 88

ways to help your kids experience big ideas, 110–111

big questions

asking better questions, 93–96

awe and intellectual humility, 103–104

awe-curiosity connection, 89–90

breaking down myths and silos, 100–101

cognitive accommodation, 88–89

making room for hobbies, 105–109

as source of awe, 10

transcendent thinking, 97–98

upside of struggle, 101–103

when you wonder, you're learning, 90–93

Big Think, interview with Keltner, 145

The Big Umbrella (Bates and Bates), 193

bird listening, 30, 31, 36

Bittersweet (Cain), 158–161, 181

Black Abstraction (painting), 66

Blackall, Sophie, 139

Blige, Mary J., 43

Bloom, Benjamin, 107

Boiger, Alexandra, 140

Booth, Leslie Barnard, 112

Borba, Michele, 106, 107, 108, 187–188

Boss, Todd, 54, 64

The Boston Globe, Snead on Ronan's "Wow," 54

The Boy Who Said Wow (Boss and Kheiriyeh), 54, 64

Braiding Sweetgrass (Kimmerer), 95

brain

art and the developing brain, 68

curiosity and the developing brain, 88, 90–91

development of middle school brain, 14

effects of exercise on, 33–34

kid's brains as hardwired for empathy, 181

mental chatter, 25–27

music and the developing brain, 46, 47–49, 50, 53, 60

nature's stimulation of, 31, 33

novelty as spurring, 34

retooling of, 101

toxic stress and the developing brain, 72

training of to notice and absorb everyday pleasures, 176

transformation of during teen years, 50, 97–98, 121, 122

brain synchrony, 117

Brainvolts (Northwestern University), 45

Brantley-Newton, Vanessa, 63

Brown, Dan, 62

Brown, Marc, 139–140

Bunner, Natalie, 123–125

Bussgang, Lynda Doctoroff, 150

C

Cain, Susan, 158–161, 181

Calhoun, Lawrence, 157

Campbell, Marcy, 192

Campoy, F. Isabel, 84

Cañas, Daniel, 164

Carson, Rachel, 17, 27

A Chair for My Mother (Williams), 193

Challenge Success (Stanford University), 12

Chamberlain, Rebecca, 68

Change Sings (Gorman and Long), 140

Chatter (Kross), 25–26

Cheavens, Jennifer, 172

Child Lab (Massachusetts), 143

childhood, slowing down of (parenting anchor), 11–12

Chin, Jason, 41

circle of life

cosmic questions, 144–145

helping kids navigate loss, 152–156

living in the moment, 142–144

picture books about, 163–165

post-traumatic growth, 156–161

as source of awe, 10

tale of two butterflies, 145–147

ways to help your kids experience the lifespan, 162–163

wisdom of elders, 147–152

Clevenger, Sharon, 149, 151, 152

coaches, what we can learn from them, 125–130

cognitive accommodation, as feature of awe, 88–89

cognitive development, theory of, 88–89

Cole Thomas, 66

collective effervescence, as source of awe, 10, 116

collective neuroscience, 116–117

Collins, Anita, 43, 48, 49

Columbia University, research about teens and science, 102

Common Sense Media, report on young people's screen time, 19–20

community, picture books about, 139–140

compassion, benefits of, 171

Comport, Sally Wern, 140

Cornell University

Lab of Ornithology, Merlin (app), 31, 36

research on nature's influence on mental health, 22

cortisol, 71–72, 142

courage, as source of awe, 170

Cregg, David, 172

Crockett, Johnson, 85

Crump, Lil, 84

Csikszentmihalyi, Mihaly, 106

curiosity

awe-curiosity connection, 89–90

impact of on learning and memory, 91

practicing radical curiosity (parenting anchor), 13–14

D

Dalaunay, Sonia, 85

Daley, Ken, 41

Damour, Lisa, 50–51, 187

Dan + Claudia Zanes, 57, 58, 59

Dancing Hands (Engle and López), 63

Daniel Tiger's Neighborhood (TV show), 152

David, Susan, 141, 167

daydreaming, benefits of, 32

De Cruz, Helen, 93

death, children's questions about, 144–145

Dell'Antonia, KJ, 119–120, 176

dePaola, Tomie, 41

Digging for Words (Kunkel and Escobar), 112

Donald in Mathmagic Land (cartoon), 100

dopamine, 51, 123

Doty, James, 171

Driscoll, Susanna, 73

Durkheim, Émile, 116

E

Each Kindness (Woodson and Lewis), 193

eclipse, awesomeness of, 17–18

Edelman, Hope, 154–155, 156, 157

Edmunds, Atticus, 53, 54

Edmunds, Tresa, 53

ekphrasis (description), 65

elders, wisdom of, 147–152

embracing PDF (Playtime, Downtime, Family time) (parenting anchor), 12–13

Emotional Agility (David), 167

The Emotional Lives of Teenagers (Damour), 50, 187

empathy, kids' brains as hardwired for, 181

Engle, Margarita, 63

Environmental Health and Preventative Medicine, Li article on forest bathing, 28

Erskine, Kathryn, 140

Every Little Thing (Marley and Brantley-Newton), 63

Expulsion from the Garden of Eden (painting), 66

The Extended Mind (Paul), 32–33

F

Fagell, Phyllis, 185, 186

Faller, Heike, 165

family activities, as creating belonging, 134–135

Fantastic Fungi (film), 36
Farmer, Ray, 76–77
"Fascinated by Nature" (video), 29
Finding Winnie (Mattick and Blackall), 139
five senses game, as way to help kids experience nature, 40
Fleming, Denise, 40
Fletcher and the Falling Leaves (Rawlinson and Beeke), 163–164
Flett, Julie, 164
flow, state of, 106
Fogelson, Marni, 63
Ford, A. G., 139
Forest Bathing (Li), 28
forest bathing (*shinrin-yoku*), 28–29
Frazee, Marla, 164
Freakonomics (podcast), quote from Green, 175

G

Garfinkle-Crowell, Suzanne, 49–50
Gee, Nancy, 142
generosity, nature and, 23–25
Gill, Nikita, 195
Gillen, Lynea, 192
The Girl Who Heard the Music (Fogelson, Teave, and Miguéns), 63
The Girl Who Thought in Pictures (Mosca and Rieley), 112
The Girl with Big, Big Questions (Lee and Souva), 112
Goal! (Javaherbin and Ford), 139
Goldstein, Evan, 92–93
The Good Life (Waldinger and Schulz), 13, 134
Good People Everywhere (Gillen and Swarner), 192
goodness
    picture books about human goodness, 192–193
    turning toward goodness, 175–177
goosebump moments, 3, 4, 5, 14, 36, 44–45, 52, 54, 59, 75, 109, 170, 178
Gordon, James S., 70

Gorman, Amanda, 140
Gottman, John, 176–177
Grandin, Temple, 112
GrandPré. Mary, 84
gratitude, 168–169
Greater Good Magazine
    Keltner article on feeling awe, 170
    Levasseur article on awe walks, 28
    on nature and awe, 24
Green, John, 175
Green, Rebecca, 112
grief, 154–156
grief dosing, 155
grief spike, 154, 155
Gruber, Matthias, 91
Guillain, Charlotte, 41
Gutiérrez, José Alberto, 112

H

Hamid, Rasha, 40
Happy Dreamer (Reynolds), 111
Harlem Grown (Hillery and Hartland), 192
Harold and the Purple Crayon (Johnson), 85
Harris, Michael, 55
Hartland, Jessie, 192
Harvard University
    Center for the Developing Child, on resilience in children, 187
    Graduate School of Education (Arts and Learning), 74
    Kennedy School, study on feelings of helplessness and hopelessness, 173–174
    Making Caring Common project, 181
    Medical School, research on gratitude, 168
    Project Zero, 81, 96
Have You Filled a Bucket Today? (McCloud and Messing), 193
Hawking, Stephen, 87, 109, 110
The Heart and the Bottle (Jeffers), 164
Hebrew SeniorLife, 150, 151
helpers
    becoming, 180–182
    finding, 173–175

Herbert, Gail, 84
Hernandez, Leeza, 62–63
Hickman, Aimee Evans, 54–55
The Hidden Life of Trees (Wohlleben), 90
Hill, Amanda Rawson, 164
Hill, Heather, 94–95
Hill, Jen, 193
Hillery, Tony, 192
hobbies, making room for, 105–109
Holzwarth, Devon, 63
Hood, Susan, 140
Hope for Cynics (Zaki), 174
Hopkin, Gerard Manley, 160
hormones. *See also* cortisol; dopamine; oxytocin
    "feel-good" hormones, 142
    stress hormones, 20, 28, 72, 142
Houdon, Jean-Antoine, 66
How to Be a Happier Parent (Dell'Antonia), 119, 176
How to Bird (Hamid), 40
How to Make a Bird (McKinley and Ottley), 85
How to Raise Kids Who Aren't A**holes (Moyer), 121, 182–183
Howell, Theresa, 84
human goodness, picture books about, 192–193
human kindness
    awesome power of one caring adult, 187–190
    becoming helpers, 180–182
    coaching tweens through the interference, 185–186
    finding helpers, 173–175
    how parents can confront the crisis of kindness, 182–183
    as number-one source of awe, 170
    in praise of "tiny kindness," 177–179
    as source of awe, 10
    turning toward goodness, 175–177
    what we know about kids, kindness, and awe, 170–172
    wonderful ways to spread kindness with kids, 191–192

Human Nature and Potentials Lab (University of Chicago), 7
Hundred (Faller and Vidali), 165
Hunt, Rachel, 177–178, 190
Hurst, Elise, 113
Hutchins, Hazel, 84

I

I Love You All the Time (Kris and Zivoin), 165
"I Wandered Lonely as a Cloud" (Wordsworth), 33
In Every Life (Frazee), 164
In the Small, Small Pond (Fleming), 40
Instagram, 35
intellectual humility, awe and, 103–104
interference, coaching tweens through, 185–186
The Invisible String (Karst and Lew-Vriethoff), 165
Isabella Stewart Gardner Museum, 79–80

J

Jackson, Ne'Kiya, 94
James, Molly, 29
James Webb Space Telescope (NASA), 26
Jatkowska, Ag, 62
Javaherbin, Mina, 139
Jayden's Impossible Garden (Mangal and Daley), 41
Jeffers, Oliver, 164
John Templeton Foundation, podcast with Keltner, 95
Johnson, Calcea, 94
Journal of the American Medical Association, study on benefits of volunteering, 182
journaling, as way to help kids experience nature, 39

K

Karst, Patrice, 165
Keats, John, 65
Keltner, Dacher, 1, 3, 4, 6–7, 9, 10, 11, 20, 36, 44, 88, 93, 95, 105, 106, 142, 145, 170

Kerstein, Lauren H., 164
Kheiriyeh, Rashin, 54, 64
Kim, Tia, 118
Kimmerer, Robin Wall, 95–96, 104
kindness. *See also* human kindness
  coaching kids toward, 185–186
  crisis of, 182–183
  as source of awe, 170
  Tiny Kindness, 177–179, 190
  wonderful ways to spread kindness with
    kids, 191–192
knowledge emotions, 89–90
Ko, Queena, 80–81
Koehler, Amy, 128–129
Kraus, Nina, 45–47, 48, 49
Kris, Deborah Farmer, 2, 7, 88, 111, 146, 165
Kross, Ethan, 25–26, 31–32
Kusama, Yayoi, 85

L

Land, Edwin, 93–94
Last Stop on Market Street (Peña and
    Robinson), 192
Learning How to Learn (Oakley and
    Sejnowski), 101
Lee, Britney Winn, 112
Leone, Raymond, 51
Levasseur, Aran, 27–28
Lewis, E. B., 193
Lew-Vriethoff, Joanne, 164, 165
Li, Qing, 28
life, circle of, wonder of, 141–165
lifespan, ways to help your kids experience
    the lifespan, 162–163
likability, as form of popularity, 123
Listen (Stocker and Holzwarth), 63
Lithgow, John, 62–63
loneliness
  defined, 115
  as public health epidemic, 115
Long, Loren, 140
Look and Be Grateful (dePaola), 41
López, Rafael, 63, 84
loss

helping kids navigate loss, 152–156
  picture books about, 163–165
Loujain Dreams of Sunflowers (Mishra-
    Newbery, Al-Hathloul, and Green), 112
Luyken, Corinna, 192
Lyons, Kelly Starling, 63

M

Ma, Yo-Yo, 44
Magic Ring (sculpture), 80
Magsamen, Susan, 70
Mainzer, Amy, 18
Making Caring Common (Harvard University),
    181
Maliekel, Lindsey Buller, 131–132, 133
Mallett, Keith, 63
Manes, Cara, 85
Mangal, Mélina, 41
Maps (Mizielińska and Mizieliński), 42
Marley, Bob, 63
Marley, Cedella, 63
Marley, Ziggy, 62
Martin, Marc, 112
Mattick, Lindsay, 139
Mattin, Ronan, 53–54, 56
Maybe Something Beautiful (Campoy,
    Howell, and López), 84
McCloud, Carol, 193
McKinlay, Meg, 85
Medical College of Wisconsin, study on
    relationship between nature and
    mental health, 22
Mehretu, Julie, 65
Memories of a Birch Tree (Cañas and Millán),
    164
mental chatter
  defined, 25
  nature and, 25–27
mental health
  art and, 70–72
  music and, 49–52
  nature, awe, and, 20–23
Merlin (app), 31, 36
Messing, David, 193

Messner, Kate, 41
Meta-Gallup, survey on loneliness, 115
Middle School Matters (Fagell), 185
Miguéns, Marta Álvarez, 63
Millán, Blanca, 164
Miller, Pat Zietlow, 193
Mindshift (TV show), 158
Mishra-Newbery, Uma, 112
Mister Rogers' Neighborhood (TV show), 152, 154
Mitchell, Jeffrey, 102–103
Mizielińska, Aleksandra, 42
Mizieliński, Daniel, 42
Monroy, Maria, 9
Montessori, Maria, 36
moon watching, as way to help kids experience nature, 39
A More Beautiful Question (Berger), 93
Morrison, Toni, 188, 189
Mosca, Julia Finley, 112
Moyer, Melinda Wenner, 120–121, 182–184
Mueller, Megan, 142
Munene, Pete, 130
Murthy, Vivek, 115
music
    and the developing brain, 46, 47–49, 50, 53, 60
    different between noise and sound (and why
        it matters), 45–49
    and mental health, 49–52
    picture books about, 62–64
    rhythm as core ingredient of, 47–48
    sensory-friendly performances, 56–59
    as source of awe, 9
    use of to connect with kids, 52–55
    ways to help your kids experience music, 61–62
The Music Advantage (Collins), 43
Music Is in Everything (Marley and Jatkowska), 62
Muth, Jon J., 140

N
NASA's James Webb Space Telescope, 26
National Geographic Kids Almanac, 111
National Institutes of Health (NIH), study on nature's influence on mental health, 22
nature
    and attention, 29–32
    benefits of, 19, 20–22
    better thinking through nature, 32–34
    as "buffer," 22
    and generosity, 23–25
    as key source of awe, 18
    and mental chatter, 25–27
    onscreen, 35–36
    picture books about, 40–42
    as source of awe, 9
    ways to help kids experience nature, 39–40
nature journaling, 39
Neal, Christopher Silas, 41
Nelson, Emily, 59–61
Netherlands, research on awe and kindness, 171
Never Play Music Right Next to the Zoo (Lithgow and Hernandez), 62–63
New Victory Theater (NYC), 131–132
The New York Times
    "A Divided America Agrees on One Thing: The Eclipse Was Awesome," 17–18
    "Taylor Swift Has Rocked My Psychiatric Practice," 49–50
Nobel, Jeremy, 71
Noguchi, Isamu, 80
Noguchi Museum, 80
noise, as compared to sound, 45–49
The Noisy Paint Box (Rosenstock and GrandPré), 84
Northwestern University, Brainvolts, 45
Noticing (Yamada and Hurst), 113
Novack, Kate, 98
NPR
    article on Silvers, 120

interview with Gee, 142
interview with Mueller, 142

O

Oakley, Barbara, 101
"Ode on a Grecian Urn" (Keats), 65
Of Sound Mind (Kraus), 45
Ohio State News, interview with Cheavens, 172
Ohio State University, study on acts of kindness, 171–172
O'Keeffe, Georgia, 66
Oliver, Mary, 195
Orozco, César, 55
Ottley, Matt, 85
Our Table (Reynolds), 139
outdoor playtime, benefits of, 33–34
Over and Under the Pond (Messner and Neal), 41
oxytocin, 121, 123, 142

P

Packs (Salyer), 140
parenting
    author's anchors of, 11–14
    as push-pull, 15
Paul, Annie Murphy, 32–33
PBS KIDS, author's description of nightly ritual, 175–176
PDF (Playtime, Downtime, Family time), embracing of (parenting anchor), 12–13
peer approval, 123–124, 186
peer groups, 121–122, 123
Peña, Matt de la, 192
Penfold, Louisa, 74, 75–76
performing arts, belonging and, 130–133
Piaget, Jean, 88
picture books
    about art, 84–85
    about belonging and community, 139–140
    about human goodness, 192–193
    about life and loss, 163–165
    about music, 62–64

about nature, 40–42
    to inspire big ideas, 111–113
Piff, Paul, 24
A Place to Be (Leesburg, Virginia), 51
Planet Earth (TV series), 35
poignancy, 147
Pope, Denise, 12
Popular (Prinstein), 121
popularity, 122–123
Porter, Tenelle, 104
post-traumatic growth, 156–161
Potts, Natalie, 82
practicing radical curiosity (parenting anchor), 13–14
Preston-Gannon, Frann, 40
Prinstein, Mitch, 121–122, 123
Project Zero (Harvard University), 81, 96

Q

question mirroring, 111
questions
    big. *See* big questions
    cosmic questions, 144–145
    what if ... questions, 111

R

Radiant Child (Steptoe), 85
radical curiosity, practicing of (parenting anchor), 13–14
Ramos, Fatinha, 85
Ransom, Hattie, 22–23
The Rashi School (Dedham, Massachusetts), 147–149
Rawlinson, Julia, 163–164
Recycled Orchestra of Paraguay, 140
Redwoods (Chin), 41
Regan, Nanette, 164
Reinhardt, Django, 55
Remembering Sundays with Grandpa (Kerstein and Regan), 164
Ren, Amber, 62
Reynolds, Peter H., 111, 139
rhythm, as core ingredient of music, 47–48
Rieley, Daniel, 112

rituals and routines
    author's family's nightly ritual, 175–176
    as creating belonging, 134–135
    Toddsgiving ritual, 184–185
Roberto, Michael, 34
Robinson, Christian, 112, 192
Rogers, Fred, 90, 119, 152, 154, 173, 181, 187, 189
Rosenstock, Barb, 84
Ross, Ivy, 70
Rutland, Ariel, 139
Rydzewski, Ryan, 90

S
Sainte-Marie, Buffie, 164
Salyer, Hannah, 140
Santomero, Angela, 152
Satellites 27 (painting), 65
Schaefer, Adam, 40
Schaefer, Lola M., 40
Schulz, Marc, 13, 134
Schwartzberg, Louie, 36
"The Science of Awe" (Allen) (Greater Good Science Center), 2–3, 89
Scientific American, article on brain synchrony, 117
screens, accessing nature through, 35–36
Sejnowski, Terrence, 101
Semioli, Mark, 127–128
sensory-friendly performances
    importance of, 56–59
    things to look for in, 58
Sexton, Anne, 65
shinrin-yoku (forest bathing), 28–29
"Shorn, treaded red" (Wadud), 65
Sierra, Judy, 139–140
silence, as part of healthy sonic diet, 47
Silvers, Lauren, 120
Silverstein, Shel, 48
Silvia, Paul, 89, 90
Sing a Song (Lyons and Mallett), 63
60 Minutes, segment on Johnson and Jackson feat, 94

slowing down childhood (parenting anchor), 11–12
Snead, David, 54
social savoring, 176
Somebody Loves You, Mr. Hatch (Spinelli and Yalowitz), 193
Something Good (Campbell and Luyken), 192
song share, 52–53
Sonia Delaunay: A Life of Color (Manes and Ramos), 85
Sorby, Sheryl, 69
sound, noise as compared to, 45–49
Souva, Jacob, 112
spatial reasoning, art and, 68–70
Spinelli, Eileen, 193
"Spring and Fall" (Hopkin), 160
Stanford University
    Center on Longevity, research on older adults being resources for children, 150
    Challenge Success, 12
    on completing creative tasks, 33
"The Starry Night" (Sexton), 65
status, as form of popularity, 123
Steptoe, Javaka, 85
Still This Love Goes On (Sainte-Marie and Flett), 164
Stocker, Shannon, 63
A Stone Is a Story (Booth and Martin), 112
Stone Soup (Muth), 140
The Street Beneath My Fee (Guillain and Zommer), 41
struggle, upside of, 101–103
Stuckey, Heather L., 71
student comments
    Alejandra, 144
    Alice, 153
    Anna, 195
    Araya, 51
    Ava, 128
    Celia, 47
    Grace, 144
    Kate, 29

Kate Novack, 98
Keira, 151
Luna Faye, 133
Marinda, 117
MJ ("Vinny") Worsley, 98–99
Naomi Hopkins, 189
Paige, 74
Riley, 179
Suzuki, Sarah, 85
Suzuki, Wendy, 33–34
Swarner, Kristina, 192
Sweeney, Linda Booth, 139
Swift, Taylor, 49–50

T

Teave, Mahani, 63
Teckentrup, Britta, 40
Tedeschi, Richard, 157
thinking, better thinking through nature, 32–34
This Art Is for the Birds (Bednarski), 84
Thomas, Vicki, 29
Thoreau, Henry David, 33
"Three Little Birds" (song), 63
Thrivers (Borba), 106
Tigner, Steve, 79
Tiny Kindness, 177–179, 190
Toddsgiving ritual, 184–185
Tracy, Bill, 126–127, 129
transcendent thinking, 97–98
Tree: A Peek-Through Picture Book (Teckentrup), 40
Twenty Questions (Barnett and Robinson), 112

U

University of California, Davis, study on curiosity, 91
University of Chicago, study of children and awe-inspiring experiences, 7
University of Southern California (USC), research on transcendent thinking, 97

Unlocking Creativity (Roberto), 34
Up in the Garden and Down in the Dirt (Messner and Neal), 41

V

Van Gogh, Vincent, 65
Vidali, Valerjo, 165
Vonnegut, Kurt, 115

W

Wadud, Asiya, 65
Waldinger, Robert, 13, 134, 135, 172
Washington Post, Leone essay on music, 51
Weinstein, Ellen, 85
Weissbourd, Richard, 181–182
what if … questions, 111
When I Draw a Panda (Bates), 84–85
When You Wonder, You're Learning (Behr and Rydzewski), 90
Wiggles, 56
Wild Symphony (Brown and Batori), 62
Willems, Mo, 62
Williams, Michelle Blouin, 94
Williams, Vera B., 193
Winfrey, Oprah, 188
Winter (sculpture), 66
Wohlleben, Peter, 90
Wolf, Dennie Palmer, 131, 132
WolfBrown, 131
Woodson, Jacqueline, 193
Woolf, Virginia, 33
Wordsworth, William, 33, 59
"The World Is Too Much with Us" (Wordsworth), 59
Worsley, MJ ("Vinny"), 98–99

Y

Yalowitz, Paul, 193
Yamada, Kobi, 113
Yang, Fan, 7, 116
Yayoi Kusama: From Here to Infinity (Suzuki and Weinstein), 85

You Have Feelings All the Time (Kris), 7, 146

You Wonder All the Time (Kris and Zivoin), 2, 88, 111

You'll Find Me (Hill and Lew-Vriethoff), 164

Your Brain on Art (Magsamen and Ross), 70

Z

Zaki, Jamil, 174–175, 176

Zaks, Laura, 184

Zanes, Dan, 59

Zivoin, Jennifer, 111, 165

Zommer, Yuval, 41

ZooZical (Sierra and Brown), 139–140

READING GUIDE

1. In the introduction, the author writes, "Awe is perhaps our most overlooked and undervalued emotion." How much did you know about awe and wonder before reading this book? As you read, did any of the benefits or sources of awe surprise you? What is the greatest source of awe in your life?

2. Think back on your childhood to a moment or two when you felt awestruck. What do you remember about that experience? Did it involve one or more of the sources of wonder described in this book (nature, music, art, big ideas, belonging, cycle of life, or human goodness)?

3. Awe researcher Dacher Keltner told the author, "How do you find awe? You allow unstructured time. How do you find awe? You wander. . . . How do you find awe? You slow things down. You allow for mystery and open questions rather than test-driven answers." In your family life, what might it look like to wander or to slow things down? In our achievement-oriented culture, how can we make more room for mystery and open-ended questions?

4. Slow Down Childhood is one of four parenting anchors described in the introduction. The other three are Embrace PDF (playtime, downtime, family time), Practice Radical Curiosity, and Become an Awe-Seeker Yourself. Which of these resonates most with you and why? Do you have any additional anchors for your parenting that you would add to this list?

5. Chapter 1: The Wonder of Nature describes many of the benefits of getting kids outdoors. And yet, in general, children today

spend less time outside than children in previous generations did. What are some practical or creative ways you can connect (or reconnect) your kids with nature? What gets in the way? Do you notice a difference in your mood or your child's mood when you spend time outside? Are there aspects of nature that reliably help you feel awe?

6. In Chapter 2: The Wonder of Music, neuroscientist Nina Kraus encourages parents to pay more attention to kids' auditory worlds. Think about how sounds—from phone alerts to blasting a favorite song in the car—affect you and your family. How can you be more intentional about managing your sonic environment?

7. In chapter 2, several stories are shared about using music to connect with kids. What are your thoughts about using music as a tool for connecting with your child? What positive musical memories do you have with your family? Has music ever helped you connect with your child or your family during more difficult moments?

8. Chapter 3: The Wonder of Art describes the *awe*some benefits of making and viewing art. What resources are available in your home and community for making, seeing, or engaging with art with your child? How might you and your child engage with art in the coming months?

9. In chapter 3, several artists and educators describe how art helps kids and teens explore the unknown, or—as one teacher put it—"leave space for not knowing." What do you think this means, and why might it be important for kids and teens?

10. Chapter 4: The Wonder of Big Ideas explores the connection between awe and learning. According to research, awe is tied to

curiosity, and curiosity about a topic improves kids' academic outcomes. What are some ways you can nurture your child's curiosity? What is sparking *your* curiosity these days?

11. As kids grow and change, so do their passions and interests. Think about a time when your child felt apathetic about or disconnected from school, an academic subject, and/or an activity that used to bring them joy. How did you help them navigate this shift? What might you do differently next time?

12. Chapter 5: The Wonder of Belonging examines children's desire to belong to something larger than themselves. Can you think of a moment when you or your child experienced "collective effervescence"—the awe that comes from being part of a group working in harmony toward a common goal? What were some of the key ingredients to that moment?

13. Kids' desire to belong can take them on an emotional roller coaster as they try to find their place socially at each stage of development. What insights from chapter 5 can help you support and guide your child in navigating these ups and downs?

14. Chapter 6: The Wonder of the Circle of Life looks at beginnings and endings. A rabbi told the author, "To shield children entirely from death and the dying process—and even the aging process—is doing them a disservice." Do you agree? How might you help your child stay connected with awe and wonder during difficult times without minimizing their grief?

15. In chapter 6, the author discusses the benefits of connecting younger and older generations. Does your family have the opportunity to interact with people from across the lifespan,

including the very young and the very old? How can you help your child forge authentic connections with people of all ages?

16. Chapter 7: The Wonder of Human Kindness notes that the most common source of awe is noticing the goodness of other people. Given the often-bleak headlines, how do you balance keeping your child informed about the world while also highlighting everyday acts of kindness and courage? What else might you do?

17. Fred Rogers's mother told him to "look for the helpers" during difficult times because "you will always find people who are helping." In what ways does your child help around your home, their school, and their community? How might you help them grow their "helper muscles"?

18. Has reading *Raising Awe-Seekers* influenced the way you think about parenting? If so, how?

19. While you were reading this book, what moments made you think, "I want to try that with my kids!" or "I need more of that in *my* life"? How might you make time for and do those things?

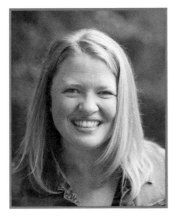

Deborah Farmer Kris is a child development expert, parent educator, and the author of the "All the Time" and "I See You" children's book series. Her bylines include *CNN*, PBS KIDS, NPR's *MindShift*, *The Washington Post*, the *Boston Globe Magazine*, and *Oprah Daily*.

Deborah spent over twenty years as a K–12 teacher and administrator and currently serves as an expert advisor for a PBS KIDS show *Carl the Collector*. Mostly, she loves sharing nuggets of practical wisdom that can help kids and families thrive.